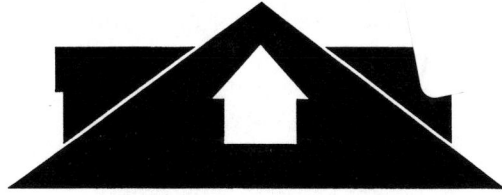

Care Homes and Dementia

Conference papers presented at Warwick in March 2000 and articles relating to care homes and dementia from the *Journal of Dementia Care*

Introduction
DR Richard Hawkins

Editor
Sue Benson

THE JOURNAL OF DEMENTIA CARE

CARE HOMES AND DEMENTIA
Conference 2000

This book draws together conference papers presented at Warwick in March 2000
and articles on related themes published in the *Journal of Dementia Care*

First published in 2001 by
Hawker Publications Ltd
13 Park House
140 Battersea Park Road
London SW11 4NB
Tel 020 7720 2108, Fax 020 7498 3023
Email hawker@hawkerpubs.demon.co.uk

British Library Cataloguing in Publication Data

A Catalogue in Publication Data

ISBN 1 874790 57 4

Designed by Andrew Chapman

Printed and bound by The Book Factory, London

Hawker Publications publishes the *Journal of Dementia Care* and *Caring Times*. For further information
please contact Hawker Publications at the address above or see our website: http://www.careinfo.org

Books published by Hawker Publications include:
Person-Centred Care. Edited by Sue Benson. £6.99.
ISBN 1 874790 54 X
Openings – Dementia Poems & Photographs. By John Killick and Carl Cordonnier. £9.99.
ISBN 1 874790 49 3. 2000.
Care to Communicate. By Jennie Powell. £16.95. ISBN 1 874790 48 5. 2000.
ASTRID – A guide to using technology within dementia care. Compiled and edited by Mary Marshall. £9.99.
ISBN 1 874790 52 3. 2000.
The Care Assistant's Guide to Working with People with Dementia.
Edited by Sue Benson. £13.50. ISBN 1 874790 37 X. 1998.
Improving Dementia Care: a resource for training and professional development.
By Buz Loveday, Tom Kitwood and Brenda Bowe. £59.99. ISBN 1 874790 38 8. 1998.
You Are Words – Dementia Poems. Edited by John Killick £6.50.
ISBN 1 874790 32 9. 1997, reprinted 2000.
Design for Dementia. Edited by Stephen Judd, Mary Marshall and Peter Phippen. £49.50.
ISBN 1 874790 35 3. 1997.
The New Culture of Dementia Care. Edited by Tom Kitwood and Sue Benson. £17.50.
ISBN 1 874790 17 5. 1995, reprinted 1997.

All books are available from Hawker Publications as above or
through reputable bookshops.

CARE HOMES &
DEMENTIA | # Contents

Contributors

CAROLE ARCHIBALD RGN is senior fieldworker at the Dementia Services Development Centre at the University of Stirling. She has worked in the field of dementia care for nearly 20 years. Her interests include activities for people with dementia, respite care, specialist dementia units and sexuality.

STEVE BONNER works with Edinvar to explore the practical use of technology to help people with special needs, including those with dementia. He has previously looked at domestic energy management in the Western Isles and worked in an advocacy role with low-income and disadvantaged households in Edinburgh.

BRENDA BOWE Dip COT is practice development manager for Anchor Trust and runs Dementia Training & Consultancy Services with Buz Loveday. Brenda qualified in Ireland in 1979 and has worked in London since 1984 specialising in elderly and dementia care. She is an associate trainer of the Bradford Dementia Group.

JAN DEWING has worked in clinical practice across a variety of settings, most recently in community hospital settings with older people and their families and with primary health care teams. She has held a variety of joint posts between trusts and universities and more recently with the RCN Institute. She became senior fellow at the RCN in 1998.

STEVE HOPKER has worked in Bradford since 1990 as a consultant psychiatrist. He is chair of the local mental health prescribing committee and has been involved in discussions regarding new drug treatments for dementia.

ANTHEA INNES worked as a part-time activities organiser in residential and nursing homes. She is now a researcher with Bradford Dementia Group.

ALISON JOHNSON is a freelance charity consultant on issues concerning older people. She was formerly Secretary of Methodist Homes for the Aged with responsibility for policy, information and research. In 1997 she visited Australia as a Winston Churchill Fellow, looking at facilities for older people with dementia.

STEPHEN JUDD PhD is chief executive of the Hammond Care Group, based in Sydney, Australia, which provides direct care services for more than 450 people. Stephen has more than 18 years' experience in the healthcare and information technology industries.

JOHN KILLICK has been writer in residence for Westminster Health Care for more than eight years, concentrating on people with dementia. He is also Research Fellow in Communication Through the Arts at the Dementia Development Services Centre, University of Stirling. He is author of *You Are Words: Dementia Poems* and *Openings*.

BUZ LOVEDAY Dip Couns runs Dementia Training & Consultancy Services with Brenda Bowe. She is an associate train-er of the Bradford Dementia Group. Together she and Brenda provide specialist dementia care services across London and the surrounding areas.

MARY MARSHALL MBE is director of the Dementia Services Development Centre at the University of Stirling. Professor Marshall has worked with and for older people for most of her career as a social worker, lecturer, researcher and voluntary organisation manager. She has written and edited several books about working with older people.

HAZEL MAY has an MA in Philosophy and Health Care and currently practices as an independent state-registered occupational therapist. She has led a number of Dementia Care Mapping projects in nursing and residential homes in addition to designing and running courses for family carers.

MARY McILWAINE is a care assistant in a dementia care home in Belfast.

SANDY PAGE works full time as deputy head of Mackintosh School of Architecture, Glasgow. He is currently involved in research into housing for elderly people and through this has been most recently involved in the *Just Another Disability* project, Glasgow '99.

LYNNE PHAIR is nursing and care management adviser at RSAS AgeCare. She has worked with older people for most of her career. She spent 16 years working in the NHS in community services for older people with mental health problems, working as a CPN and team leader.

JACKIE POOL is a state-registered consultant occupational therapist in dementia care. Her practice, Dementia Concern, provides training and clinical services in the NHS, social services and the private sector; she has also developed the website www.DementiaConcern.com, which provides an online advisory service for people with dementia and their carers.

JENNIE POWELL PhD is qualified in Human Communication and Neuropsychology. She is currently working as a clinician and researcher with the Memory Team, Llandough Hospital, Cardiff which provides diagnosis and appropriate long-term psychosocial management for people with memory impairment and dementia.

DAVID SHEARD works full time as a dementia care consultant/trainer for Care Matters. He is a training consultant with the Alzheimer's Society and has worked as an associate consultant with the Dementia Services Development Centre, University of Stirling. He works extensively throughout the UK, promoting a holistic approach to dementia care.

SALLY STEWART is an architect and tutor at the Mackintosh School of Architecture, Glasgow. As a member of the panel of architects working on a series of customised residential environments for people with dementia, she is currently working on a series of publications documenting the *Just Another Disability* project.

Introduction

*T*he client profile in care homes has changed enormously in the last five years. 'Frail' elderly people are almost never placed in homes, and even those with significant physical disabilities are becoming rarer.

Instead homes are increasingly populated with people who have some degree of confusion, memory loss or dementia. Estimates suggest anything from 50 to 70 per cent of residents in non-specialist homes may be affected. And of course there are now numerous specialist homes, either converted or purpose built.

The knowledge gap in many of these homes is huge, although there are some very notable exceptions who provide first-class care. It takes much more than just goodwill to work with and care for people with dementia successfully, in a way that makes the most of all opportunities for enhancing well-being and independence, as well as helping to lessen agitation, distress and challenging behaviour.

This book has therefore arisen out of the considerable need for specialist care of people with dementia in a residential setting. It is based on a very successful conference held by the *Journal of Dementia Care*, and supplemented by key articles selected from the Journal over the last few years. It is not intended to be comprehensive. Instead it addresses key areas and issues which experienced personnel feel are the topics most likely to be helpful to staff in a care home setting.

The Journal and I would like to thank the many people who have contributed in whatever form, either as clients or staff.

DR RICHARD HAWKINS
Editor-in-chief, *Caring Times* and *Journal of Dementia Care*

CHAPTER ONE | Person-centred care in care homes

LYNNE PHAIR

Nursing and care management adviser, RSAS Agecare

Person-centred care is different from other models of care that have been promoted over the past decade. Models such as primary nursing, individualised care and holistic care are systems for those that deliver care. For people with dementia who live in a care home it is not enough for just the care staff to work in a certain way. Everyone involved in the life of that person, from the chef to the administrator, needs to follow a way of life, a philosophy and have an attitude that is person-centred, and that is why this approach is fundamentally different.

When Kitwood and Bredin (1992) first developed this model, it was for some an innovation and for others confirmation and a theoretical framework for this approach to care (Phair & Good 1989). Person-centred care is as relevant for managers and commissioners of services as it is for care staff. To implement it successfully in a care home however, it is important to understand the theory and Kitwood's belief system which underpins it.

Traditional culture

The traditional view care staff have held about people who have dementia, is that they, the care staff, are basically sound, competent, kind people, while people with dementia are neurologically impaired and thus damaged and deficient. We are given skills to manage their illness. We are given skills to manage their challenging behaviour and to live the way that we have decided in our institution. We do not have any problems, we are here to manage their problems (Kitwood 1993a,d; 1995d).

The new culture

Today we realise that a more helpful perspective is that the gap between care staff and those with dementia is actually very narrow. Everyone has some deficiencies, and everyone has problems. The difference is that people with dementia may lose the ability to hide their feelings; they express their emotions in a more immediate, authentic way. Care staff on the other hand have the ability to protect themselves by denial and collusion, and can put on a veneer of politeness (Kitwood 1993a,d; 1995d).

Principles of person-centred care

Personhood

The underlying principle of person-centred care is that the person with dementia is respected as a fellow human being who happens to have some special needs. Kitwood identified what makes someone a person and what enables that person to feel valued (well-being) and the damage that can be done by other humans to a person causing them distress (ill-being) (Kitwood 1997c).

We accord an individual the status of a person when we acknowledge:
• his unique make up as an individual
• his place in the human group
• his needs
• his value simply because he is a human being
• his rights.

To support this, four key elements are added:
• **personal worth** – we must feel wanted by somebody
• **agency** – we can have an effect on the world around us (we can make things happen, and make choices)
• **social confidence** – we can trust the people we are with
• **hope** – we must always feel that things can be better.

Personhood and personal worth are elements of being that everybody would aspire to, regardless of what disease labels they have attached to them.

What is dementia?

Kitwood and Bredin have shown that dementia is not just a disease causing cognitive impairment. The impact of that disease can be affected by a combination of aspects of the person's life; if that is not acknowledged, the care given cannot truly assist the whole person. These aspects are:
• **personality** – the person's character and how that influences their view of the world
• **biography** – the person's life path, with all the major events and losses that have taken place
• **health** – the person's state of health, including acute and chronic physical and psychiatric illnesses
• **neurological impairment** – the dementia itself
• **social psychology** – the effect of their current social environment on a person's life.

Key elements

In caring for people with dementia, we have to ensure that every aspect of the person's self is cared for and supported. As well as a high standard of physical care and nutrition, the psychological care of the person is crucial.

The principles of person-centred care must focus around the need to support the person, ensuring their emotional well-being. However well furnished the home is, or indeed how well the person is 'cleaned and fed', if attention is not paid to their emotional well-being the person with dementia is not being valued as a whole person. To this end, the whole life of the home should focus on the six key principles set out below. These principles of respect for the person with dementia should form the cornerstones of life in a care home:

- **holding** – both physical and psychological, supporting them either with a hug, holding their hand, or giving emotional support by showing you understand their feelings
- **validation** – acknowledging the person's experience and emotion is real; denying their experience denies their feelings
- **facilitation** – enabling a person to do what they can for themself (staff should just do the bits they can't)
- **celebration** – the care staff and older person enjoy life together, working in partnership and as equals
- **stimulation** – the pleasurable stimulation of the senses; the environment should smell, look and sound encouraging, and the person with dementia encouraged to enjoy that
- **relaxation** – the atmosphere care staff work in should be unrushed, with care staff working calmly alongside residents, and no one under unnecessary pressure.

Malignant social psychology

The routines and attitudes of the home can do untold damage to the well being of the person with dementia. As a way of life, a home which follows the philosophy of Person Centred Care should be acutely aware of the potential harm words and actions can have on a person's self-esteem. Kitwood identified 17 aspects or actions which damage the personhood, lower the self-esteem and foster feelings of failure in the person with dementia (Kitwood 1997).

The person with dementia may not be able to express why they feel hurt or upset (they may have forgotten what was said or done to them) but the negative feeling can remain, just as a positive feeling will remain after the person has been helped or praised, even though the words are forgotten. One negative comment or action may not cause the person damage, but if the culture of the care home is one of negativeness, reprimand or task allocation, repetitive negative approaches will cause long term harm to the person with dementia. That person may then respond with behaviour traditionally viewed as 'challenging'. The person may express their frustration as anger, aggression or by wanting to leave the home. Alternatively, the person may turn inwards and become

so demoralised that they see no point in trying to care for themselves, and so become more dependent in their physical care needs.

The 17 components of malignant social psychology can occur mildly or severely; the damage to the person could be instant or incremental, but as with people who do not have dementia, if a person is continuously downtrodden or criticised it will affect their self-esteem, their confidence and eventually their self-belief.

- treachery – the use of dishonesty or deception to obtain compliance
- disempowerment – the care staff doing something for a person that they are quite capable of doing for themselves
- infantilisation -implying that the person has the mentality of a child and speaking to them in a condescending manner
- condemnation – blaming or accusing the person.
- intimidation – the use of threats, abuse of the power of the care staff
- objectification – talking about the person, or dealing with them as if they are an object
- stigmatisation – intimating that they are different, that there is a 'them and us' divide between residnets and staff
- outpacing – giving information too quickly, not bearing in mind the needs of the person
- invalidation – ignoring the feeling demonstrated or expressed by the person
- banishment – removing the person, physically or psychologically
- ignoring – talking with another in the presence of a person as if they are not there
- imposition – forcing a person to do something
- withholding – refusing to respond if a person asks for help
- accusation – blaming a person for failures that arise due to their lack of ability
- disruption – disturbing a person suddenly without respect
- mockery – making fun of a person's unusual behaviour
- disparagement – telling the person they are failing.

Developing person-centred care in a care home

I hope this brief introduction to the philosophy and practice of person-centred care will be enough to encourage managers and supervisors to begin by examining what really happens in the care home. And to look from the position of a spectator at the life of the residents.

Sitting in the lounge of the care home and just watching life from the residents' point of view can enable the observer to see whether they are being cared for as *people* who happen to have dementia; or are they being cared for as 'Doris the Lewybody and Bert the Alzheimer's'? (Kitwood 1997)

Honesty of the observer and an hour to sit and watch life is all that is required for this exercise – together with an understanding of the basic principles of person-centred care set out here.

The observer may see:
- a momentary hug from a care assistant to a resident
- a compliment on their choice of clothes
- a passing chat with a resident as the staff do their work
- a conversation between two residents resulting in them sharing a biscuit
- the general assistant asking a resident to help lay the table, or arrange the flowers, smelling them and touching them.

Or, sadly, the observer may see:
- residents calling for assistance and being ignored
- residents being moved with a hoist without being told what is happening to them
- residents asking for a cup of tea and being told 'it's not time'
- residents standing up to walk and repeatedly being sat down by staff
- residents being chastised for 'making a mess' with a pot plant they were looking at.

Once the observer has begun to get a flavour of life in the care home lounge, they can begin to help other staff to examine their own practice and attitudes towards the residents. The first and most important principle to establish among all the staff in the home is that they really understand and believe that the staff and the residents are equals, and that any discriminatory language or action is dispelled. Once this belief system is established, with reinforced education and training, the home can become an environment that will encompass person-centred care. The philosophy has to be a total belief system. Recent research has identified that just training staff in isolation is not enough to ensure person-centred care works (Woods, Lintern & Phair 2000). The organisation, support staff and care staff must ensure that time, equipment and resources are available to support the direct care staff in this philosophy. Organisational issues and time for communication are also vital if care is going to be delivered in this way.

Staff at every level have a role to play in the development of person-centred care.

Senior managers and commissioners have to ensure the organisation underpins the approach by:
- good recruitment procedure
- attitude-focused induction programmes
- philosophy-focused training and education
- ensuring time for staff communication
- ensuring supervisory support is available
- ensuring regular review of the philosophy of the home and how that is being lived
- that care equipment is available and appropriate
- that furniture and furnishings are positive – ie of good quality, not necessarily plastic or damage resistant – and that recreational equipment is available
- that staff are employed who are actively encouraged to engage the residents in the life of the home.

Direct and non-direct care workers should ensure that:
- the residents are known to staff as people, by obtaining life histories and ensuring appropriate activity is offered
- that the routine of the home is truly resident-focused and not home-focused
- that they do inform temporary or new staff of the philosophy and that negative attitudes are unacceptable
- that appropriate risk assessments are employed with the principle of empowerment and managed risk rather than negative paternalism
- residents are encouraged to help around the home, with staff from any department within the limits of safety and their ability
- that residents are welcomed into anyone's office at any time; unless the information being handled is confidential.

Inspectors of homes should ensure that:
- there is a method in the inspection process to enable examination of the impact of the philosophy on the resident
- that staff are encouraged to examine positive risk taking and enablement of residents rights
- that the inspectors themselves understand the principles of person centred care.

For those involved in the development of new services and new buildings, the principles of good design (Judd, Marshall, Phippen 1998) should be central to any project. High quality interior fabrics and decoration should be used to ensure a positive physical environment; but also resources should be made available for the real development of the philosophy and culture of the home. If this is not undertaken and continuously reinforced the initial investment will be fruitless (Woods, Lintern & Phair 2000a,b).

The investment in the building will also be lessened as the technology, interior decoration and design will only be used to their full potential if the culture and philosophy enable it to work (Phair 1999).

Person-centred care should be a way of life for everyone in the care environment. Its impact and progress can be measured formally by using Dementia Care Mapping (Bradford Dementia Group 1999), but it can be implemented and should be used for every older person with dementia, as the best and most appropriate model of care.

References

Bradford Dementia Group (1999) *Evaluating Dementia Care: DCM Method*. Seventh edition. University of Bradford.

Judd S, Marshall M, Phippen P (1998) *Design for Dementia*. Hawker Publications, London.

Kitwood T, Bredin K (1992) Towards a theory of dementia care, personhood and well-being. *Ageing and Society* 12 269-87.

Kitwood T (1993) Towards a theory of Dementia care: the interpersonal process. *Ageing and Society* 13 51-67.

Kitwood T (1995) Cultures of care, tradition and change in Kitwood T, Benson S (eds) *The New Culture of Dementia Care.* Hawker Publications, London.

Kitwood T (1997a) The uniqueness of persons with dementia in Marshall M (ed), *State of the art in dementia care.* CPA, London

Kitwood T (1997b) *Dementia Reconsidered.* Open University, Buckinghamshire.

Phair L, Good E (1989) People, not patients. *Nursing Times* June 7 Vol 8523, 42-44.

Phair L (1999) Does the design of the environment help or hinder the care of older people with advanced dementia? Unpublished Florence Nightingale Scholarship Report

Woods B, Lintern T, Phair L (2000a) Before and after training: a case study of intervention. *Journal of Dementia Care* 8(1) 15-17.

Woods B, Lintern T, Phair L (2000b) Training is not enough to change care practice. *Journal of Dementia Care* 8(2) 15-16.

Useful address

Dementia Care Mapping, Bradford Dementia Group, School of Health Studies, Unity Building, 25 Trinity Road, Bradford BD5 OBB.

CHAPTER TWO | Communication: a matter of life and death of the mind

JOHN KILLICK

Poet, author and writer in residence for Westminster Health Care and for the Dementia Services Development Centre, Stirling

My title is a bold assertion. I don't intend to present scientific arguments for its truth (in any case I am not qualified to do so). Rather, I hope to convince by conviction and circumstantial evidence that the proposition is worth serious consideration. To begin with, there are a number of premises with which, I hope, we can all agree:
● Dementia results in communication difficulties for the person with the disease.
● These difficulties present problems for the person who would communicate with them.
● Failure to make progress in overcoming these can have serious consequences for the caring process:
- possible sense of isolation for the person with dementia;
- disempowerment of that person;
- the tendency for others to deny personhood to them.

The concept of personhood has been defined by Tom Kitwood in a number of articles and books. He rejects the mindset of 'a set of deficits, damages and problem behaviours, awaiting systematic assessment and careful management' (Kitwood 1993) and the medical model from which they derive in favour of a holistic approach, seeing the dementia as a complex interaction between physical disease, personality, life history and social relationships. He speaks of a 'malignant social psychology' which effectively prevents the individual from functioning as an individual.

From my own experience as a writer working in institutional settings I can give an example of this. In the early days, my presence in nursing homes was seen with a good deal of incomprehension. (Things have improved a great deal lately, and perhaps my role has in a small way helped to influence this change.)

One morning I went into a mental health unit and sat in a lounge waiting to make contact with someone. A lady near me indicated that she wished to talk, and I began not only to engage in an absorbing conversation with Mrs Andrews but also (with her permission) to make a written record of it. After about twenty minutes a care assistant came over.

'Why are you speaking to Mrs Andrews?' she asked.

'Because she spoke to me, she is a most interesting person, and I have already made a record of our conversation,' I answered. 'There must be some mistake,

Mr Killick. Mrs Andrews has nothing to say for herself,' was her astonishing reply.

An essential beginning

It seems to me self-evident that communication must take pride of place in our design and delivery of care for persons with dementia. With the present state of knowledge about causes and cures, we have to adopt a pragmatic approach to alleviating the situation of individuals in the here-and-now, and without consulting them, without listening very hard to what they are trying to tell us, we can't have any notion of what their needs may be.

Mary Marshall's book *State of the Art in Dementia Care* (1997) devotes no fewer than nine chapters to communication, and there are very few of its other chapters which do not touch on the subject.

I work as a writer for Westminster Health Care, a major provider of nursing home care throughout Britain, and many of the texts of conversations end up as poems. A few years ago I completed a piece of work at Stirling University, funded by the Linbury Trust, turning some of these poems into a book (Killick 1997a). Here is an example, a lady speaking:

Life is a bit of a strain,
in view of what is to come.
Sometimes I feel embarrassed
talking to anybody, even you.
You don't really like to burden other people
with your problems.

I have been a strict person.
What people and children do now
is completely different. Any beauty
or grace has been desecrated.
The circle of life is shot away.

I want to thank you for listening.
You see, you are words.
Words can make or break you.
Sometimes people don't listen,
they give you words back,
and they're all broken, patched up.

But will you permit me to say
that you have the stillness of silence,
that listens, and lasts.

When she says 'you are words' she may be paying a personal tribute but she is also talking about all of us.

She shows an awareness of the future and what it may have in store, a reluctance to trouble others, consciousness of the passage of time and social change, and gratitude for time and trouble taken. But above all she shows an overwhelming awareness of the importance of communication. She sees it as a two-way process, and expresses a great deal of pain over what she perceives as the failings of others in understanding and valuing what she has to say. The next voice is that of a man:

> It's a good idea,
> this writing it down;
> it's got a bit of merit.
> It's tantamount to saying
> you're speaking from your memory all the while.
>
> In the War I went around
> and I saw nothing that wasn't
> a waste of time and life.
> The door opened to dust
> and I thought it might be me tomorrow.
>
> Such unselfish lives
> just putting themselves last
> in all walks. No bitterness
> or anguish, all loving-kindness.
> Now the evening is coming to its close for me.
>
> You don't see your family
> much now: like a carrier-bag
> on your back, one way or another.
> But you can't barge it or dish it –
> all of it was everwell.

This shows many of the same characteristics as the previous poem. In addition, there is an attempt at an evaluation of his life, and also a sense of preparedness, of resignation. Here is a third voice, a lady again:

> I have a problem.
> I have a house on either side of the road,
> but I only have a room in one of them.
> How do I cross the busy road?
> And what happens if I break down in the middle?
>
> I have another problem.
> I've spilt something on my skirt.
> There's nothing there?
> Are you sure there's nothing there?
> Well it must have been in another room.
> Well it must have been in the other house.
> Well it must have been another skirt.
>
> And I have a problem about kindness.
> A lot of those who come round here
> are not interested in being kind to others.

> Kind is the only thing one can do here.
> It is all there is that can help.
> I don't try to be it.
> You shouldn't have to try to be kind.

This piece comprises the articulation of worries. They are on different levels: we may think that the middle worry is comparatively trivial, but what right have we to say that? Certainly there is nothing trivial about the worry that she might break down in the middle of the road; and there is more than one meaning of the phrase 'break down'. This lady is concentrating on survival, and the last verse could surely serve as a text to be inscribed over many workplaces.

Here is a fourth piece, another lady. She has problems with language, and in her behaviour exhibits the phenomenon known as 'wandering':

> I'm just going to see what's round the corner...
>
> I've lived here twenty-five weeks in the city,
> up and down the language, twice up and down...
>
> I'd better just have another look...
>
> I'll tell you if you can understand the language.
> And I'm talking, talking, talking all the time...
>
> I'm just off to see if it's changed at all...
>
> I didn't know if you would understand,
> with you living on the other side...
>
> I'll just see if it's all right over there...
>
> Young girls wearing white on the other side
> of their dress, getting married...
>
> I'll just see if I can get far enough along...

This is far more confused, and her words seem to mirror her actions. She mixes up thoughts and images and misses connections. Yet she is just as concerned with communication as the other speakers, and in that extraordinary pair of lines in which she speaks of me 'living on the other side' seems to reveal a profound understanding of her situation.

The time to listen

A final example, which can also serve to illustrate the phenomenon of variability of response. I had tried to work with this lady on the previous day but had hardly been able to obtain single-word answers from her. The onus had all been on me to question and supply possible replies. But now, my role was almost exclusively a listening one, and she knew exactly what she wished to say:

I'm forstering. I'm becoming more... well put it this way: nothing would stop me talking if I could find something to talk about. I've been a secretary for twenty years, so where did I go wrong?

People haven't got time to talk to me now because it takes such a long time. I've never been an over-volulous person. I'm feeling I'm getting more silent. I feel that no one wants to bother with me any more.

My mind, my whole sphere of life, is full. I was very fond of my life. It seems that I'm leaving it more and more. Oh dear, it isn't fair when your heart wants to remember!

I often wonder why people bother with people like us. I could have reeled off for what you are doing. It's a life-story. It's the biography of the person you are writing about. It's me.

This is a mental home, you know. Most of the people living here need looking after. And if I was truthful I would say that that includes me.

This short piece, extracted from a much longer text, reveals so much. Not the least of its remarkable qualities is the awareness it shows of my role as a writer. But if I had to find one word to sum up what these five pieces (along with many others I could have quoted) have in common, that word would be 'insight'.

Language is the barrier

I profoundly believe, from my experience of working with hundreds of people at all stages of the disease over several years, that this quality – insight – remains, and the barrier which they (and we) have to fight against is the language in which to embody it.

With many residents in the homes where I work, language has almost won. Many relatives say of their silent loved ones 'There's nothing there any more'. But occasionally when I have been sitting with these silent ones I have been privileged to witness 'the clouds part' (Killick 1997b) and I have been vouchsafed words which interpret the muteness:

I think about it all. Everything. I pick up what I want and what I don't I leave. I sift it and the rest goes down.

The past, I think a lot about it. I'm thinking when... I'm not saying... I can't tell people things.

To return to my title, I want to make two final points. The urgency placed on communication comes in so many cases from the person with dementia. A glance back through my texts here will furnish a number of examples.

Then there is the lady who asked me:

Would you please give me back my personality?

To me she hadn't lost it, but it was her perception that she had – and she was desperate to hang on to what language she had left. It was the same lady who said:

I want to get to the point where it's a case of a matter of course. What is this lump of matter if you can't make sense of it?

Moral commitment

Tom Kitwood in his book *Dementia Reconsidered* wrote the following passage: 'Dementia will always have a deeply tragic aspect, both for those who are affected and for those who are close to them. There is, however, a vast difference between a tragedy, in which persons are actively involved and morally committed, and a blind and hopeless submission to fate.' (Kitwood 1997)

In the absence of any certainty about the true role of communication in relation to insight in persons with dementia, I suggest we adopt the position of behaving as if communication is a matter of the life and death of the mind. It is surely the only truly 'actively involved and morally committed' course of action open to us.

References

Killick J (1997a) *You are words: dementia poems.* Hawker Publications, London.
Killick J (1997b) When the clouds part. *Journal of Dementia Care* 5(1) 24.
Kitwood T (1993) Discover the person, not the disease. *Journal of Dementia Care* I(I) 16-17.
Kitwood T (1997) *Dementia Reconsidered.* Open University Press, Milton Keynes.
Marshall M (ed) (1997) *State of the Art in Dementia Care.* Centre for Policy on Ageing, London.
• This chapter first appeared as an article in the *Journal of Dementia Care* 5(5) 14-15.

CHAPTER THREE | Helping caregivers understand communication problems of people with dementia

JENNIE POWELL
Memory team, Llandough Hospital, Cardiff

*I*t is well recognised that people with dementia have difficulty with communication. This paper will describe a 'model' of communication that tries to explain what may be happening for the person with dementia when communication breaks down. It is suggested that an understanding of this model of communication can allow professional caregivers help people with dementia overcome some of the communication difficulties experienced.

Communication involves the transmission of ideas. Most commonly we think of communication as the transmission of ideas from person to person when ideas may be communicated non-verbally (Fig 1), with words (Fig 2) or with a combination of non-verbal and verbal communication (Fig 3).

In reality, the communication process is much broader than this and involves the transmission of ideas from environment to person as well. Moment to moment we are 'checking' our surroundings to determine how we should react and respond. When all is well we feel at ease and can relax (Fig 4).

Sometimes the idea we receive from the environment is that something is threatening and requires an immediate response. For example, an approaching car speeding around the bend communicates to us that we should terminate our plan to cross the road.

At other times the brain may misinterpret the envi-

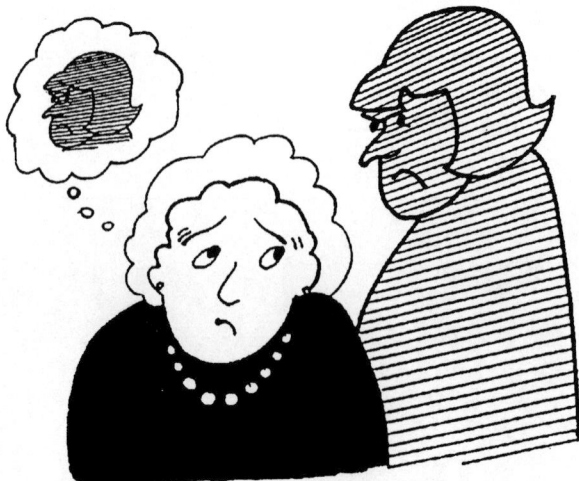

Fig 1: Communication of ideas from person to person non-verbally: 'I don't think she like me'

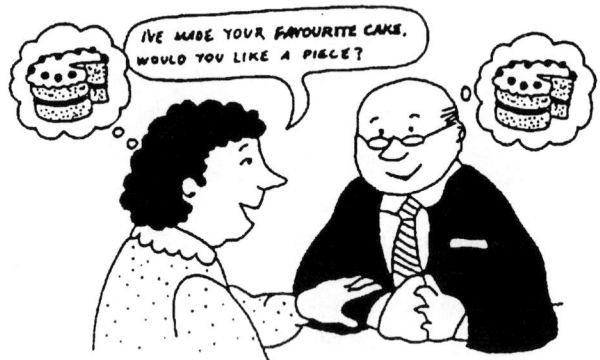

Fig 2: Communication of ideas from person to person using words

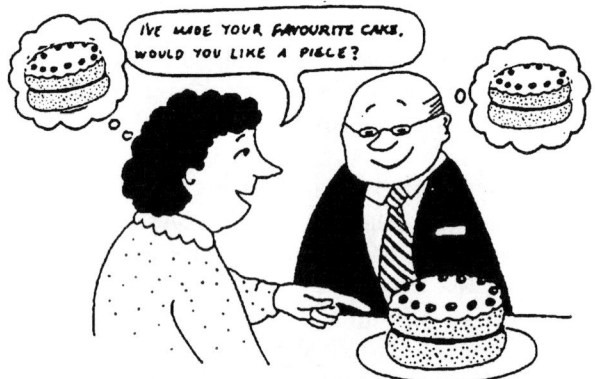

Fig 3: Communication of ideas from person to person non-verbally and with words

ronment and get the wrong idea as in Fig 5 where the scarf is perceived as a snake and the jacket seems to have a face. This sort of misinterpretation can happen to any of us, but usually it occurs just for a split second before logic and reasoning skills 'click in', correct the misinterpretation and adjust the idea.

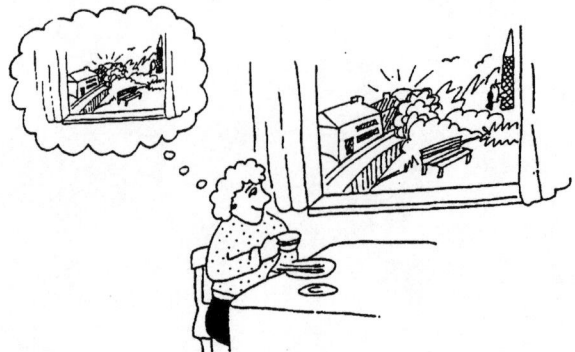

Fig 4: Communication of ideas from environment to person

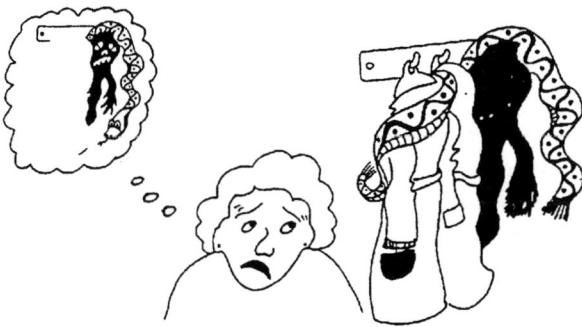

Fig 5: Misinterpretation of the environment

What then are 'ideas'? Ideas can be thought of as constructed from mind images stored in the long-term memory systems of the brain. We use thousands of mind images every day to think, to make decisions and to survive.

The basic type of mind images are those we create for objects and concepts in the world around us. For example, if asked to think about an apple, we would create a set of images in the mind of how it looks, feels, tastes, smells, sounds like when bitten and so on (Fig 6). These images form the semantic memory system of the brain, the store of knowledge we all share about the world.

How do concepts become stored in the brain's semantic memory in the first place? The semantic memory stores of the newborn infant are waiting to be filled with images from the world around. Ideas are absorbed as the world is explored by touching, shaking, sucking and so on. Gradually ideas and concepts of the environment are established to create the semantic memory store. New ideas and concepts can be added at any time in life, for example an adult learning what a passion fruit is would

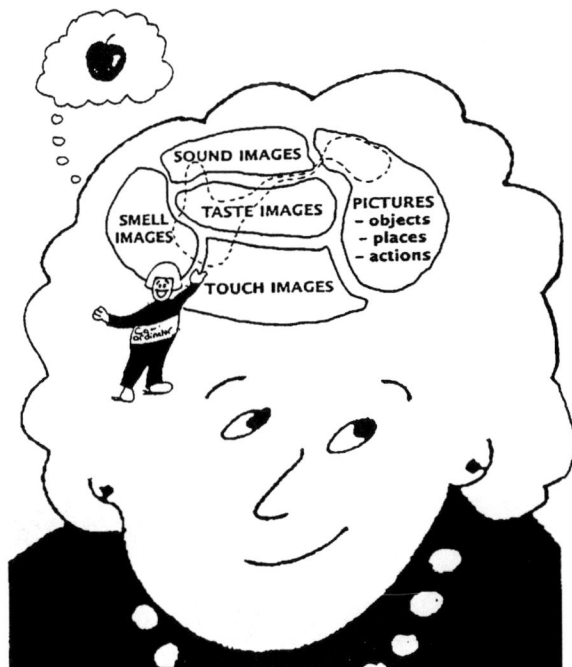

Fig 6: Hypothetical model of semantic memory

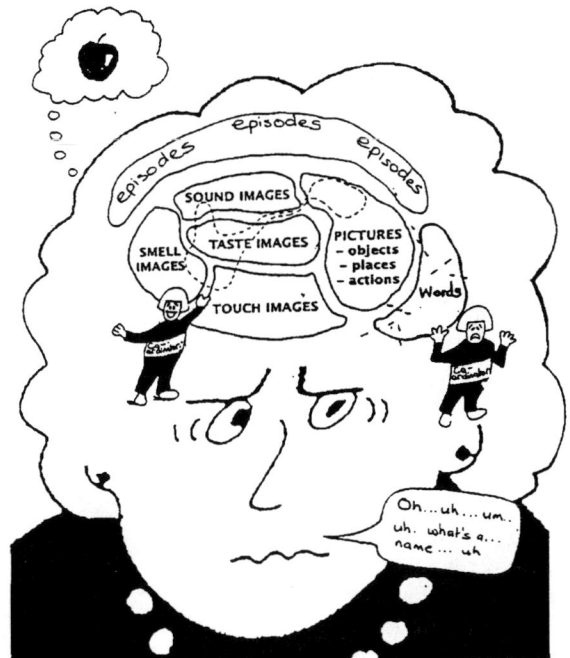

Fig 7: Breakdown of communication due to difficulty with using words (dysphasia)

do so by seeing, touching, tasting and so on just as he did for more common fruits like apples and oranges when a child.

Another type of mind image is created from events or episodes we have experienced.

These events and episodes form an episodic memory store in the brain. Episodic memory probably uses semantic memory mind images as 'building blocks'. For example, if you try to think about the last time you ate strawberries, the mind image of the episode of you sitting in your garden last summer eating strawberries would probably be created with semantic memory images of strawberries, summer and garden but with your own personal images of those concepts interwoven to form an episodic memory unique to you.

Finally, what about words? Words are stored in a mental dictionary known as lexical memory. Words are labels that describe concepts and episodes in semantic and episodic memory. Without semantic and episodic memory, words would be meaningless – think about listening to a foreign language of which you have no knowledge. Words allow us to organise ideas, to pull them into consciousness and move them around in our mind more easily.

The number of ideas and concepts we need to add to semantic memory is huge in infancy but relatively small in adulthood. The same is true for words – in infancy new words are constantly added to the lexical memory store, whereas this happens only occasionally in adulthood. With episodic memory the story is very different – as adults, new events or episodes are added to episodic memory many times every day.

When someone just has a problem with words, this is known as dysphasia (Fig 7). When dysphasia occurs in isolation, it usually is the result of a relatively confined

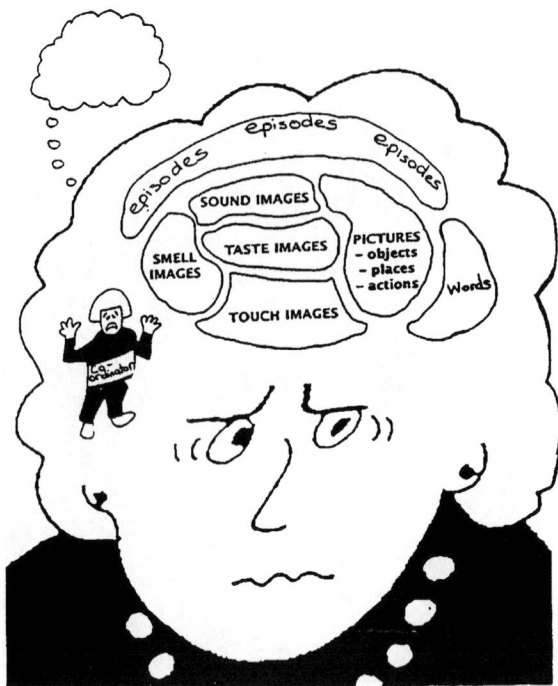

Fig 8: Breakdown of communication in dementia: difficulty activating images and ideas stored in the brain without prompting

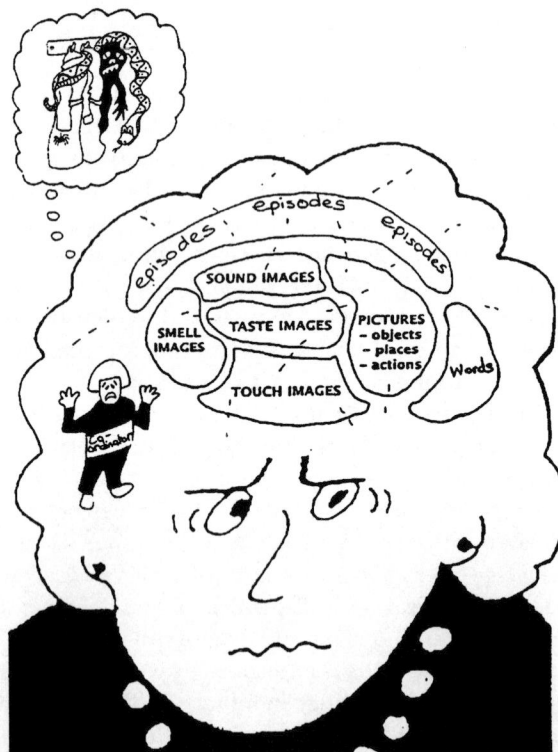

Fig 9: Breakdown of communication in dementia: difficulty organising and making sense of images that do form

brain lesion, for example following a stroke in the lexical memory area of the brain.

People with dementia can have problems with words, but for most people with dementia, communication is impaired for a much broader reason than simply diffi-

culty with words. In early dementia, the main problem affecting communication is memory impairment. This causes problems with adding new information to the memory stores. The person has difficulty adding new life event images to episodic memory, new concept images to semantic memory and new words to lexical memory. Typical consequences are, forgetting what has just happened, difficulty remembering where things have been put, forgetting appointments, forgetting the names of new grandchildren and so on. The difficulty with adding new life events to episodic memory has most impact because this needs to happen many times every day, whereas as adults only occasionally do we need to learn new concepts and words.

As dementia progresses, the person has more and more difficulty adding new memories. In addition, the person has difficulty activating images and ideas stored in the brain without prompting (Fig 8), difficulty organising and making sense of images that do form (Fig 9) and parts of images/episodes previously stored are lost (Fig 10). The difficulty with adding new images, activating them and making sense of them leads to difficulty with thinking, reasoning and making decisions.

The problem with reasoning and making decisions shows up in many ways in day to life. For example, the person may be thirsty but have difficulty activating images in the mind and so has no idea what to do about the feeling of thirst (Fig 11). She may have difficulty organising and making sense of images that do form and so be unable make a decision about which type of drink to have (Fig 12). Or she may have lost parts of images and be unable to even begin to think about what to drink (Fig 13).

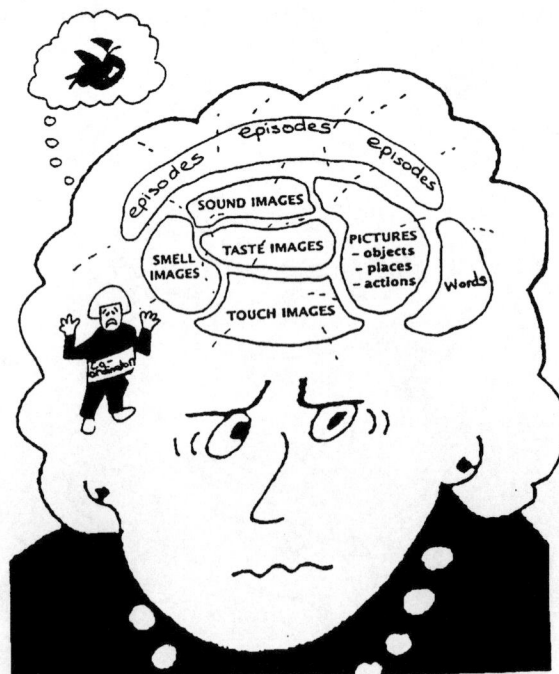

Fig 10: Breakdown of communication in dementia: parts of images/episodes previously stored are lost

Many of the difficulties with communication experienced by the person with dementia can be explained in terms of this imagery-based model of communication. Thinking about why a particular problem occurs is the first step towards learning what to do to minimise the problem. Caregivers can be taught about images in the brain by asking them to think of all the things that come into their head when they think about an apple for example. They can then be asked to imagine what it would be like if the wrong images, or no images, or mixed up images came into the head instead. Once the idea of 'mind images' is understood, carers can begin to reason out for themselves why the the person they care for reacts or responds in a particular way. This can be empowering for carers and can help them to help the person with dementia more effectively. Ideas for helping caregivers develop a problem solving approach based on the model of communication described in this chapter can be found in the book *Care to Communicate.**

The CLIPPER care plan

The person with more severe dementia will have difficulty initiating activities and interacting with others. He is unlikely to be able to help himself to even the simple pleasures of life, such as a walk in the garden or a favourite drink. In the same way he may be unable to avoid what is unpleasant for him, such as bathwater so deep it frightens him or constant pop-music in the background.

In more severe dementia, the whole quality of the person's life can depend entirely on the carer. If we fail to try to understand the unique needs of each person, we can seriously damage well-being.

The person with dementia has the right to lead as full and active a life as his illness will allow. However, it is vital that stimulation offered is appropriate both in terms of type of stimulation and amount.

The carer needs to develop the skill of interpreting the person's non-verbal messages. Watching the person's facial expressions, eye contact and body language and listening to his emotional tone of voice may help you to learn what he does and does not enjoy.

Remember also that the appropriate stimulation for an individual may be very basic – perhaps even as simple as holding someone's hand. Simple levels of stimulation such as using a soothing voice or a friendly smile can be incorporated creatively into daily care activities.

You may find it useful to record your impressions of the person's likes and dislikes in a structured way. The Cardiff Lifestyle Improvement Profile for People in Extended Residential Care (CLIPPER)* has been designed with this in mind. Its aim is to help caregivers improve quality of life, and it was designed to be used in a long-term care setting.

The CLIPPER considers 41 activities that could occur during a typical day. Caregivers note which activities occur, how often, and how the person seems to feel about

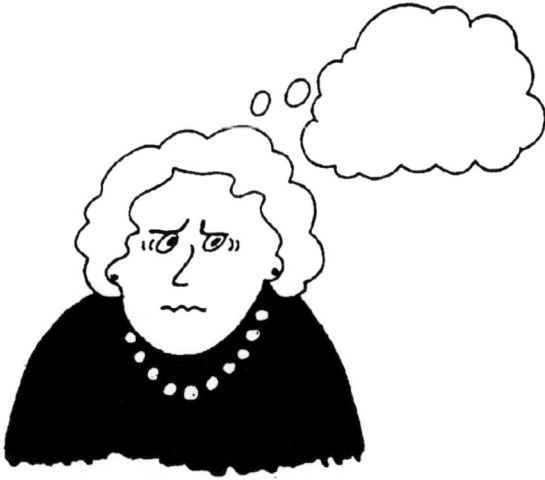

Fig 11: Difficulty activating images and ideas stored in the brain without prompting makes it difficult to know what to do about the feeling of thirst.

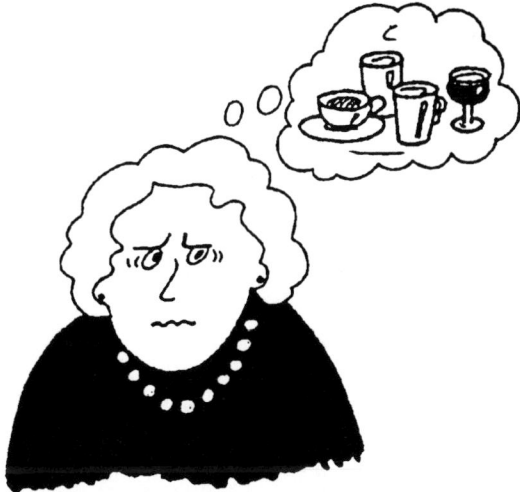

Fig 12: Difficulty organising and making sense of images that do form can make it hard to make a decision about what to drink.

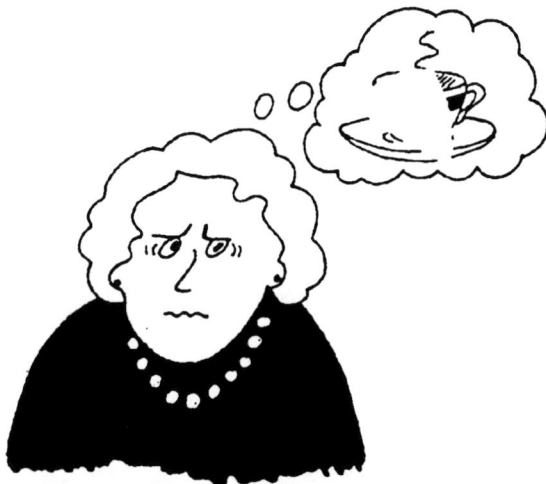

Fig 13: Parts of images previously stored in the brain are lost making it hard to even begin to make decisions.

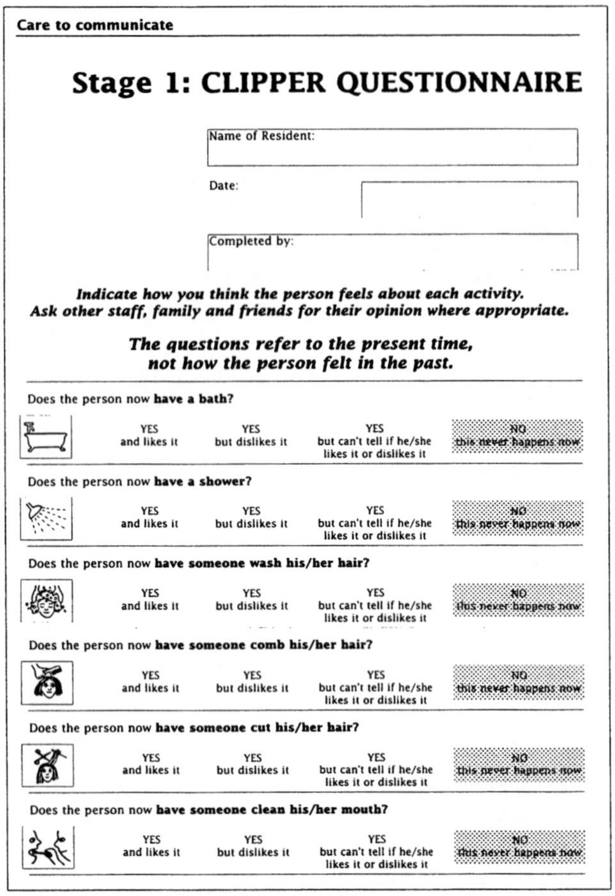

Fig 14: The first page of the CLIPPER questionnaire.

each activity. The activities are grouped into eight categories: touch and movement; watching and listening; tasting and smelling; people and pets; activities alone or one-to-one; group activities; outdoor activities; and trips, visits etc. Some activities are more passive while others encourage the person to be more actively involved. This allows a care plan carefully to be tailored so as to create the best possible quality of life for each individual.

The caregiver begins by noting which of the 41 activities occur and how the person seems to feel about each activity. For example, to the question, 'Does the person now have a bath?', the caregiver should circle one of the following: YES and likes it; YES but dislikes it; YES but can't tell if he/she likes it or dislikes it; NO this never happens.

To answer the question, the caregiver will need to consider the person's verbal and non-verbal reactions. The opinions of other staff, family and friends should also be sought where appropriate. This will give an overall impression of well-being or displeasure when the person is having a bath.

Once the caregiver has answered the same question for all 41 activities, the answers are transferred to the CLIPPER worksheet.

In the first column of the worksheet, activities that are liked are ticked. The second column documents activities that are disliked. The third column shows the 'can't tell' activities, ie those activities for which it is impossible to tell how the individual feels. The fourth column shows

activities that never happen. When the worksheet is completed, it gives a visual summary or profile of the person's daily life.

The caregiver then thinks about possible changes that could be made to make life more enjoyable. Others involved in the person's care should be asked for their ideas too, including family and friends. Ideas for changes are noted on the worksheet.

In stage 3 of the CLIPPER programme, changes that are to be tried are recorded on a formal plan and a review date is set. Caregivers and family aim to try as many of the planned changes as possible before the review. The review is usually set for 1-3 months later.

For example, Mr H has been noted to dislike having a bath. On discussion with his wife, staff thought that he may be embarrassed. The plan was to ask Mrs H to bath her husband once or twice a week. It was felt that this would also help Mrs H who had only recently given up the total care of her husband.

Staff knew that he had previously been a keen musician, but Mr H did not seem to respond to music any more. In this case the plan was:
● To find out from Mr H's family what music he liked.
● To ask family to bring in tapes.
● To encourage Mr H to use his personal stereo.

Stage 4 of the CLIPPER programme is the review. This looks at whether the changes seem to have improved the person's quality of life. For each activity, the caregiver and others involved in the person's care answer the questions below:
● Were the changes to this activity tried? YES; NO.
● Did the changes to the activity at any time improve his/her quality of life? YES; NO; Don't Know; None Tried.
● Overall, are the changes to the activity improving his/her quality of life now? YES; NO; Don't Know; None Tried.

To answer these questions, carers will need to consider the person's verbal and non-verbal responses to the changes and the overall appearance of pleasure or displeasure as a result of the changes. The whole cycle can then be repeated and a few months later the CLIPPER PLAN is reviewed to see which changes have taken place and the effects on quality of life.

The CLIPPER does not claim to be doing anything new. It is just a tool to help caregivers think about what is happening for an individual. This ensures that all possibilities for change are considered and that the best possible quality of life is achieved.

*Care to Communicate is published by Hawker Publications (ISBN 1-874790-48-5). The book includes a full, photocopiable set of CLIPPER planning sheets.

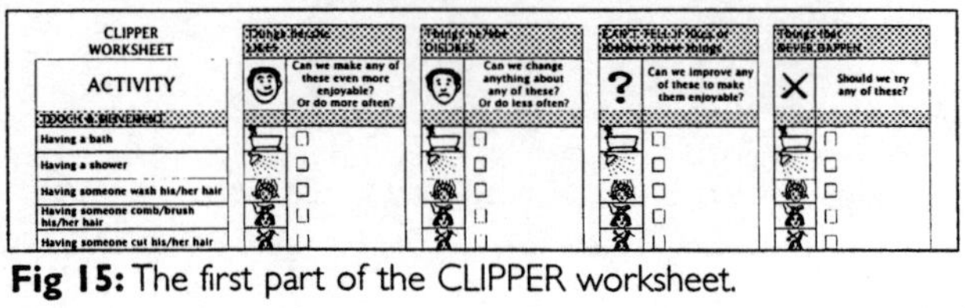

Fig 15: The first part of the CLIPPER worksheet.

CHAPTER FOUR | Rights and risk: making them compatible

DAVID SHEARD
Independent dementia care consultant

*B*alancing risks and rights in dementia care is a complex issue, but I would argue that the emphasis at present has moved too far towards risk prevention. Greater protection for the rights of people with dementia is needed, as a foundation stone of person-centred care alongside any risk management approaches.

I'd like to start with a riddle. Professor Bumble is getting on in years, and growing forgetful. On the way to a lecture one day, he went through a red light and turned down a one-way street in the wrong direction. A policeman observed the scene but did nothing about it. How could Professor Bumble get away with such behaviour?

To analyse this riddle, the risks within this situation may well be assessed as follows:
- Professor Bumble is not recognising road signs and general road safety.
- Professor Bumble is at risk of causing an accident.
- Professor Bumble is at risk of getting lost and not turning up for work.

And the rights within this situation may well be seen as follows:
- Professor Bumble has the right to continue to be productive and to engage in work.
- Professor Bumble has the right to get to work as he chooses.
- Others have the right to expect Professor Bumble to observe the Highway Code.

However, perhaps most importantly, Professor Bumble has the right not to be misunderstood: the answer to the riddle is that Professor Bumble was walking. What I want to suggest with this analogy is that perhaps we have moved to an over-emphasis on risk prevention in relation to people with dementia, when we should be promoting their rights.

Risk in dementia care

Managers providing dementia care services are having to take account of complex health and safety legislation, the need for professional risk assessments, risk taking and risk management policies. In the future, if government guidance is implemented on the extension of powers covering vulnerable adults, they will also be faced with a new Continuing Power of Attorney.

Current approaches to risk management arise from different influences in relation to duty of care, paternalism, fear of litigation and current care management approaches in the way in which assessments are undertaken. However if one contrasts this with the current state of affairs on rights, this area is far from developed. In this country we have a poor record on rights promotion compared to the USA or Europe. While the USA has a Bill of Rights within its constitution, and Europe has for some years received protection through the European Court of Human Rights, only in autumn 2000 has UK legislation established European Law in this area.

European rights

How many people in the UK can list the rights established in the Human Rights Act taken from the European Convention on Human Rights?

The first right established in legislation is introductory – a general obligation to respect human rights. This is followed in detail by specific rights, including:
- The right to life
- The right to prohibition of torture
- The right to liberty and security
- The right to prohibition of slavery and forced labour
- The right to a fair trial
- The right to no punishment without law
- The right to respect for private and family life
- The right to freedom of thought, conscience and religion
- The right to freedom of expression
- The right to freedom of assembly and association
- The right to marry
- The right to an effective remedy when rights are violated by a person in an official capacity
- The right to prohibition of discrimination
- The right to prohibition of abuse of rights

The history of rights establishment in the UK is that marginalised groups have had to fight for their rights to be enshrined in law. Too often the UK has worked on the basis that all its citizens have rights, only for groups to find they have not – be it women who have had to fight for the right to vote, black people to fight for the right not to be discriminated against or gay people to fight against homophobia. So do people with dementia need specific dementia care rights? The current state of dementia care in the UK would suggest they do; basic human rights have not been sufficient for them to receive appropriate quality of dementia care services.

So, if in running your dementia care service you have

CARE HOMES AND DEMENTIA

risk management policies and risk assessment procedures, do you also have a set of dementia specific rights against which your service can be measured? This I believe this is a foundation stone of person-centred care which is in danger of being overlooked.

Risk taking principles

So how can a service create an appropriate balance between rights and risks in providing good quality dementia care? Consider an example: Mr Sheard, who has dementia, is taken outside by you (a care worker) for a walk to prevent him feeling 'trapped in' within your service. He hits a passer by. Are you liable? This situation raises serious ethical issues about risk taking and risk assessment. Had a risk assessment already identified this as a potential hazard? What strategies had been considered and were care workers aware of these in terms of prevention? Was the care worker acting with the authority of the manager and an agreed care plan? What might be the consequences if Mr Sheard is not taken outside and might the risks be greater to himself and others?

I acted as a consultant to the Alzheimer's Society in their production of an appropriate risk assessment policy document. We established that there was a need to establish risk taking principles which would guide staff

in such a situation. The risk taking principles which have been adopted are set out in the box below left.

The Alzheimer's Society will later in the year be publishing their Risk Assessment Pack. This aims to be a practical guide, and will comprise the following sections:

1. Why a guide?
2. Person-centred approach to care – risk assessment as part of positive care.
3. Legal context.
4. Risk taking principles in dementia care.
5. Developing your Risk Assessment process.
6. Case studies and examples.
7. Implementing in different care settings.

Dementia specific rights

If an appropriate framework and balance is to be achieved in implementing risk assessment approaches, this framework should also include a set of dementia specific rights to match the above risk taking principles.

An initial good reference point in formulating a set of dementia specific rights can be drawn from *The Best Friends Approach to Alzheimer's Care* (Bell & Troxel 1997).

I suggest an adapted version of their set of dementia specific rights, as in the box below:

Risk taking principles

1. Every person has an individual personality, a history, likes and dislikes, skills and abilities and a huge variety of experience.
2. Care services for people with dementia must be provided in a way that individually recognises and builds on the person's strengths and abilities and maintains their independence.
3. Those whose mental powers are failing or have failed need, in every way, to be treated as a person just as we ourselves would like to be treated.
4. Care services for people with dementia must be provided in a way which preserves dignity and treats people with respect, offers choice and safeguards privacy.
5. Care services must have a strong emphasis on carers using their expertise and experience to improve the care that is offered.
6. The risk taking of ordinary life is necessary for people with dementia to experience continuing growth and development.
7. It is the responsibility of staff members to promote new experiences and opportunities which inevitably introduce an added element of risk.
8. People with dementia retain the rights they have always had, including choice and control over their own lives (though this brings a degree of risk.
9. The task of care services is not to eliminate risks but to determine which risks are acceptable. This should be done in conjunction with all parties concerned and without being over-protective or negligent.
10. Services will adopt a policy of measured risk taking. Risk taking will be considered in detail and a series of records kept of all views held, decisions taken, subsequent actions and an evaluation.

Rights of the person with dementia

1. To have a clear diagnosis and to be informed of this if I wish.
2. To have appropriate ongoing comprehensive medical and social care irrespective of my disability.
3. To exercise choice including the right to refuse or to have representation.
4. To have my adulthood respected even if engaging in childlike activity.
5. To have expressed feelings taken seriously.
6. To be free from psychotropic medication if possible but to have unconditional access and opportunity to be considered for new drug therapies.
7. To live in an environment which is personalised and gives feelings of being in control, inner safety, familiarity and well being.
8. To have the opportunity to enjoy and the choice to participate in personally meaningful activities on a daily basis.
9. To be given the opportunity to have social and physical contact and to participate and contribute to the wider community.
10. To be given the opportunity to be outdoors on a regular basis.
11. To be with others who demonstrate respect for an individual and their life history, taking into account race, sexuality, gender, culture and religion.
12. To be cared for by individuals who are well trained in good practice in dementia care and who demonstrate and promote this.

A folk tale from Pakistan

Consider this Pakistani folk tale originally presented at the Eighth National Alzheimer's Disease Education Conference in California (source unknown). An ancient grandmother lived with her daughter and grandson. As she grew frail and feeble, instead of being a help around the house, she became a constant trial. She broke plates and cups, lost knives and spilled water. One day, exasperated because the old woman had broken another precious plate, the daughter sent the grandson to buy his grandmother a wooden plate.

The boy hesitated because he knew a wooden plate would humiliate his grandmother. But his mother insisted, so off he went. He returned bringing not one, but two wooden plates.

'I only asked you to buy one,' his mother said. 'Didn't you hear me?'

'Yes', said the boy, 'but I bought the second one so there would be one for you when you get old.'

What do you want when *you* get old – a risk-focused service, a rights-focused service, or an approach which adopts a balance? Without addressing the rights of people with dementia we assign them to a minority position in society. Surely the future must be to attempt to provide services which balance compatible person-centred care rights and risk approaches.

References

Human Rights Act and Introduction/Study Guide (2000). Human Rights Unit Helpdesk, Home Office, 50 Queen Anne's Gate, London SW1H 9AT.

Bell V, Troxel D (1997) *The Best Friends Approach to Alzheimer's Care*. Health Professions Press. Baltimore, Maryland.

Alzheimer's Society. *A Practical Guide to Risk Assessment*. In press.

CHAPTER FIVE | An ethical approach for well-being in dementia care

HAZEL MAY
Independent occupational therapist, consultant and trainer

Why do we need to call what we do in our work with people who have dementia and their carers "an approach"? Certainly in the past there seems to have been little requirement for those involved in day-to-day caring to refer to any particular approach. However, it has been absence of such a requirement, in my view, that has formed a major part of what Tom Kitwood so dramatically termed the "malignant social psychology" (Kitwood 1990) within which countless people with dementia have lived and died.

Thankfully, times have moved forward along with our awareness and social conscience. The way we behave with and care for people who have dementia matters. Indeed, we aim to do more than provide care in this day and age, we want to improve wellbeing for the person who has dementia.

I think there are a number of reasons why consciously and openly adopting an approach is a good idea. First of all, because "we" are paid for – either from taxpayers money or directly from the person's own resources (some people sell their house these days to pay for care). There are expectations therefore by those who pay that the wellbeing of the person being cared for is paramount. This is to say, there is an expectation that "we" know what to do in order to promote and sustain well being. In a sense then, it isn't only what we do that is being paid for, it is *why* and *how* we do it. The *why* and *how* do require us to refer to some kind of rationale or approach.

As an example, think of your dentist. You don't simply buy a filling when you visit him. You buy his role as carer for you and your teeth in general. You trust him to make decisions in your best interests. For some people it will be a good thing to have a filling, for others it will be unnecessary, painful and perhaps even dangerous. You trust him not to impose unnecessary and painful treatments on you but to select the right treatments for the overall and long term good health of (you and) your teeth. He wants to look after your teeth because he values you as human being and believes that you need and deserve to live your life happily and comfortably.

Now that the concept of purchasing health and social care has become a reality and also because the status of

elderly people generally (particularly in relation to their spending power) has gained strength, we in the field of dementia care will be more under the spotlight. Increasingly will be expected to justify what we do in the same way that more traditional health and social care workers (dentists for example) do. The dentist justifies giving an injection because it prevents pain, which allows him to mend a tooth. The reason he relieves pain to mend a tooth is because of the social values we all hold in society about human beings: that (for example) they have a right to enjoy their world (we need teeth to enjoy!). The dentist's therapeutic intervention (giving an injection) is necessary to achieve his therapeutic aim (to repair a tooth) which serves a social value (that human beings should enjoy their world). This rationale ensures responsible or ethical practice.

Surely, the person with dementia is entitled to the same responsible practice. If so, then we must check that our **therapeutic interventions** (for example playing catch with a big beach ball in the lounge) are justified by **therapeutic aims** (for example with the ball, the aim might be to bring about person to person eye contact, essential for engagement with the outside world) which in turn reflect our **social values** about persons who have dementia (that they are people and therefore need eye contact, physical contact and movement to survive as such). This rationale is shown below in Fig 1.

What seems to have happened, in relation to the use of occupation in dementia care, is a tendency for off-the-shelf

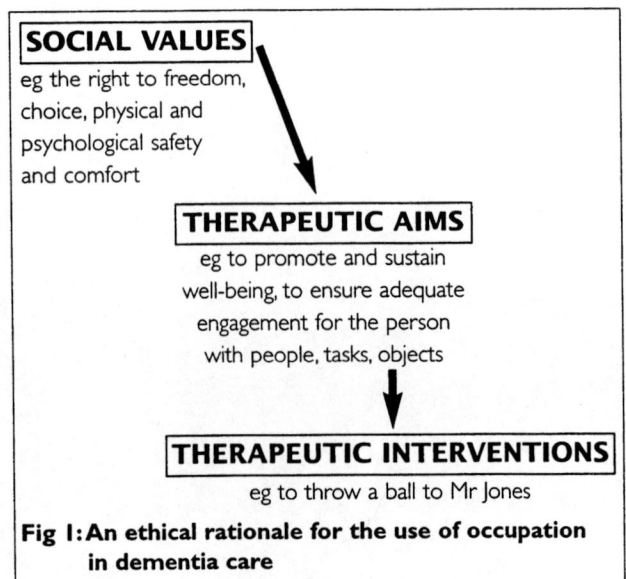

SOCIAL VALUES
eg the right to freedom, choice, physical and psychological safety and comfort

THERAPEUTIC AIMS
eg to promote and sustain well-being, to ensure adequate engagement for the person with people, tasks, objects

THERAPEUTIC INTERVENTIONS
eg to throw a ball to Mr Jones

Fig 1: An ethical rationale for the use of occupation in dementia care

purchasing of interventions without reference to the whole care role; and this is just as hit and miss for the person with dementia as it would be for a person needing dental care and getting a filled tooth which he may or may not need.

In the many hours of dementia care mapping that I have done over the years, I have repeatedly seen people with dementia on the receiving end of such hit and miss interventions. A quiz in the lounge perhaps, where only one or two people are actually engaging with the game while the rest sleep or try to escape from the group because it is uncomfortable for them. Or a "singalong" where many are enjoying it but one poor soul in the corner, who is weeping and covering her ears, is overlooked. These are well-intentioned interventions but they lack the backing of an approach or a rationale.

I believe that a good approach in dementia care should draw from two fundamental things; the occupational capacity of each individual and the impact that the intervention is having on the wellbeing of the individual.

Occupational capacity

It isn't helpful or feasible for the knowledge about occupation and how dementia alters a person's capacity to engage in occupation to remain exclusively within the occupational therapy profession. A good profession solves problems for the society it serves, and so this knowledge needs to be made usable by all in the field of dementia care; we are all concerned with and involved in the occupational life of people who have dementia. It is often our failure to understand each person's unique occupational capacity that leads to approaches which can lead to ill-being; the man who can't dress himself being told to "hurry along"; the lady feeling small and childlike as a well meaning carer brushes her hair for her when she can quite easily manage herself.

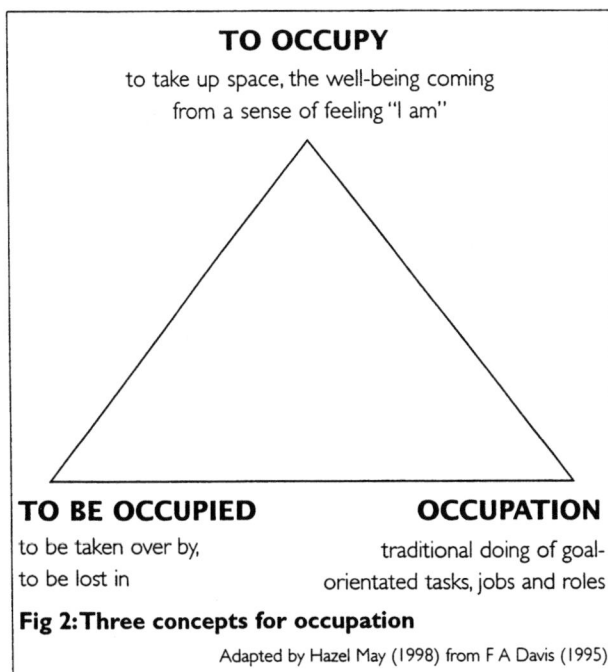

TO OCCUPY

to take up space, the well-being coming
from a sense of feeling "I am"

TO BE OCCUPIED　　　　　　　　**OCCUPATION**

to be taken over by,　　　　　　　traditional doing of goal-
to be lost in　　　　　　　　　　orientated tasks, jobs and roles

Fig 2: Three concepts for occupation

Adapted by Hazel May (1998) from F A Davis (1995)

A broader view of occupation

Historically, people who have dementia have been cared for in rehabilitative and/or mental illness services. Occupational therapists in these settings have been very concerned with independence and in using occupation to improve independence. There are problems with the carry over of this practice into dementia care. Striving for independence can undermine well-being because the concept of occupation in these fields is largely task/goal orientated (May 1998). For a person to engage in this kind of occupation, certain cognitive abilities are required. These include the ability to hold a goal in the memory; to sequence together a number of steps and to note the effect of what is being done, to name but a few. The person who has dementia is likely to lack the capacity to operate like this.

A broader view of occupation can open doors for those of us who wish to nurture an occupational existence for the person with dementia.

Consider the three different modes of occupation shown opposite in Fig 2. Within this broader view, there is the possibility of an occupational existence for all.

Mrs Morgan, who has mild dementia, continues to engage in *Occupation* by shopping for familiar items in her local store. For Mr Hiscock, who has more severe cognitive difficulties, repeated wiping of the table in the corner of the ward offers him the opportunity *To be occupied* – to become lost in what he is doing for a while. Mrs Arnold is confined to bed but is able *To occupy* the space she is in; her well-being is maintained during times when the staff help her to engage in touching, feeling, tasting, seeing.

Using a developmental approach

If occupation is to achieve a therapeutic aim (to result in well-being) for the person who has dementia, the intervention must be pitched at the right level. Expecting a person to make tea, get dressed or play Monopoly when they simply can't will not lead to well-being. Similarly, attempting to throw a ball to a person may cause ill-being if the person feels that this is childish or silly.

Using knowledge we have from the research of others into how human beings develop from being able only to respond to physical stimulation (a baby), to being able to move around (a toddler), to being able to use objects to achieve tasks (a small child) has been invaluable to a number of therapists in the field of dementia care.

Claudia Kay Allen, an American Occupational Therapist adapted Developmental Theory to propose that we might understand dementia within a framework of different levels of cognitive functioning (Allen *et al* 1992). These levels mirror the cognitive developmental levels from birth to adulthood.

Using Allen's model has helped me to develop a better understanding of cognitive capacity. In particular, I find it invaluable to assess the following key aspects of how the person relates to objects:

1. GRASP

Can the person grasp objects? This is different from what I term "primitive grasping" which is grabbing/clutching to stay upright or to put food in the mouth. This is simply an assessment of whether the person can freely and easily pick up items from the surrounding environment. If the person seems unable to do this, then it will not be therapeutic to expect the person to engage in activities that require grasping. Therapeutic interventions will need to be sensory or postural in nature. For example, rocking, licking/sucking/tasting, seeing, hearing, touching.

2. DISTINGUISH OBJECTS

Can the person work with more than one item at a time? This can be observed at meal times. If the person seems to struggle with using cutlery, they may be unable to distinguish objects. In this case, therapeutic interventions should involve grasping and repetitive actions such as wiping, stroking, rubbing...in other words "playing" with different types of object one at a time.

3. SUSTAINING ACTIONS

Can the person keep going with an action? Perhaps they potter and fiddle with whatever objects they have access to. If this is the case, it is likely that the person lacks the capacity to sustain actions on objects. The therapeutic intervention should encourage and allow pottering and fiddling!

4. NOTING EFFECTS

Can the person note the effects of what they do? This is often evident in the quality of what the person does. If the peeled potato has little patches of peel remaining, or the washed up plates have marks on them, it is likely that the person is unable to note the effects of what they do and therapeutic interventions should be thought through with this in mind.

The idea in this approach is that a person needs to be able to grasp objects before they can distinguish objects, before they can sustain action and so on.

Pitching occupation

The most common modes of occupation for people who have dementia within Allen's framework are:
• Goal directed
• Manual
• Postural

For those in the early stages of dementia who can grasp objects, distinguish objects, sustain their action on objects and note the effects of what they do, **goal directed activity** will be attractive. The person will want to engage in simple, routine, familiar occupations such as washing up or vacuuming. Card games, board games and such like will be enjoyable and achievable.

Manual activity is less demanding. Here, the person can be occupied in single step or repetitive activity without having to achieve any particular goal. The "being lost in/taken over by" occupational experience (see triangle above) comes into its own at this stage and in the postural stage (below). If the person can grasp and differentiate objects, they will feel comfortable in this kind of occupation. Wiping tables, sweeping, playing catch are examples of manual activity.

In the later stages of dementia, it seems that grasping objects and picking them up becomes difficult, and the person seems to lack the drive to engage with objects. At this stage, it is thought, the person is living a life of **postural activity** where staying upright and moving around are the main occupation. Therapeutic interventions at this stage should support this occupational existence. Pushing chairs around, waving arms and legs, rolling and rocking are all examples of postural occupation. At this level, the person will respond particularly well to physical contact and sensory stimulation.

There is so much knowledge already available to us in the dementia field about the human condition and how we evolve and develop as individuals and as a species.

The person with dementia presents us with a very real and very raw human being and I believe that we can make enormous strides forward by using what we already know about ourselves as human beings and adapting this knowledge in our work. I have found developmental theory coupled with the concept of wellbeing invaluable sources of knowledge. This provides, I believe, a good starting point for working towards a more ethical approach to dementia care in which therapeutic interventions can be clearly justified and explained through their link with the therapeutic aim of well-being.

References
Allen CK, Earhart CA, Blue T (1992) *Occupational Therapy Goals for the Physically and Cognitively Disabled* The American Occupational Therapy Association, Inc. Rockville MD.
Kitwood T (1990) The dialectics of dementia: With particular reference to Alzheimer's Disease. *Ageing and Society* 10 177-196.
May H (1998) Striving for competence can undermine wellbeing. *Journal of Dementia Care* March/April 1998 20–22.

A boost to confidence and well-being

In the course of training care assistants in residential homes across the UK, I was struck by the inconsistent approach taken by the many different staff and visitors who came into contact with people with dementia. In 1998 I produced the list below as a handout, which is now used to brief all nurses, doctors, care workers, agency staff, students, clergy, domestic staff, visitors and volunteers. It has had an immediate positive impact on both well-being of residents and confidence and job satisfaction of staff and I am happy for others to use it in care homes and similar settings. – Hazel May

Dementia Care Guidelines

At *(insert name of home)*, people who have dementia are regarded as having special needs. Although individual care plans are made for each person, there are some general approaches that can improve well-being for these residents. Staff working at this home are asked to adopt the following approaches with people who have dementia:

1. Eye contact should be made every time you provide care or come into contact with the person who has dementia.

2. Your non-verbal communication is very important; it can make the person with dementia feel safe if managed well. Your facial expression should be relaxed and friendly, your body posture non-threatening. For example, avoid towering over the person, and use gentle touch wherever you can. The tone of your voice is important too: it helps if you can talk calmly, honestly and at a relaxed pace.

3. "Outpacing" the person with dementia can cause him/her to experience feelings of ill-being. Even if you are in a hurry, try to slow down to the resident's pace. If you are feeding or dressing someone, please do so in a relaxed way.

4. Approaching the person from the front and at eye level will reduce the likelihood of the person lashing out. Our observations at this home suggest that people lash out when their personal space is invaded without any warning. Sometimes, people who have dementia do not recognise people/objects that are outside their immediate visual field.

5. Hand objects to the person at eye level and within six inches. Name the object and, if necessary, place the person's hand on the object to help them start off the action (eg drinking tea, brushing hair).

6. Whenever you can, adopt a running commentary. This simply means talking out loud to the person about what has just happened and what is about to happen. For example: "Phyllis, I'm glad you enjoyed your breakfast. We're all going upstairs now to sit in the lounge."

7. Please do not talk to other staff about residents while you are working. This is considered bad practice at this home. We prefer staff to include residents in these conversations, eg: "Phyllis, Rose and I are just talking about what a bad night you had. Do you feel tired?"

8. The person's well-being is most important. Please consider this before you step in. For example, if a resident is clearly enjoying a meal and managing perfectly well with the wrong cutlery or just with his/her fingers, it might be best not to interfere.

9. It is important to validate the person's feelings whenever you can. Try not to get into a disagreement about facts. For example, if a resident says they are hungry and that they haven't had their breakfast, you might reply, "I'm sorry you're hungry, it's a couple of hours now until lunch time, shall I go and find you a banana or a biscuit to tide you over?" Or, "Yes, I can see why that picture looks like Ashton Keynes to you. When did you last go there?"

10. Finally, please try and make a special effort with the quieter residents. Often these people are not demanding and they are at risk of being starved of human contact through the day. A brief "Hello" or short chat can make an enormous difference to their well-being. If the person can't speak, try and stroke their hand and make warm, reassuring eye contact at least once or twice during your shift.

CHAPTER SIX | Challenge or opportunity: why do we find some behaviours difficult?

JACKIE POOL

Independent occupational therapist, consultant and trainer

*E*ven in today's more informed culture of dementia care, we still refer to some behaviours as 'challenging'. This term seems to bring with it a connotation of blame: the person is being deliberately difficult by acting in some way with the malicious intent of causing distress to another. Care staff report that they feel that the behaviour of a person with dementia is challenging when they find it difficult to work with that person. There are several factors influencing who staff find it difficult to work with: if staff feel unsupported; dislike of the work or the person; have too heavy a workload; or lack the training and understanding of the situation. Staff can very quickly begin to equate the behaviour with the person and begin to view the person with dementia as difficult. Innes (1998) found that the way staff see the behaviour determines whether the person with dementia is labelled as difficult and a 'trouble maker' or as harmless. Care home staff particularly rate behaviours as difficult if they disrupt routines, create more work, or upset other residents. Residents who are viewed as not co-operating with staff are also often labelled as difficult.

Labelling

How does this labelling come about? There are two main ways it can happen. First, when a person with dementia carries out an action or behaviour, the caregiver attributes meaning to this and applies this label to the person (fig.1). In the second instance, the label already exists so that when the person with dementia carries out an action or behaviour, caregivers attribute meaning based on what they already know about the person and his or her behaviour. In this way the label is reinforced (fig 2). In both these scenarios it is apparent that the caregivers' understanding of the behaviour will influence their attribution of meaning and therefore any resulting label.

One of the principles of person-centred care is that all behaviours are viewed as messages that we should strive to understand. Some behaviours are seen as expressions of ill-being because of an unmet emotional or physical need. For example, a person who is repeatedly asking questions about where they are or what is the time of day,

is likely to be feeling anxious and insecure. Alternatively, the person with dementia may not be in a state of ill-being; they might be behaving in a way that is successfully meeting their need. However, this means of meeting the need may be unacceptable to or misunderstood by others. An example of this may be someone with dementia happily meeting a need for sexual gratification but doing so through masturbation in a public place.

When a label has been applied to a person's behaviour it can often be the case that other behaviours are then also placed under this heading and the label becomes further reinforced. To take the earlier example of sexual disinhibition, each time that person reaches out to touch another, or adjusts their own clothing, the potential for labelling that behaviour as sexually disinhibited is magnified because of the existing label. Therefore if a behaviour is to be understood and the need underlying it is to be met in a way that is acceptable to all involved, we first need to be certain of what exactly that behaviour is.

Defining the behaviour

McShane (1994) stated that we need to first define the simple atoms of the behaviour and suggested that in order to really understand something we need to take it to bits and study the parts. He uses the example of 'wan-

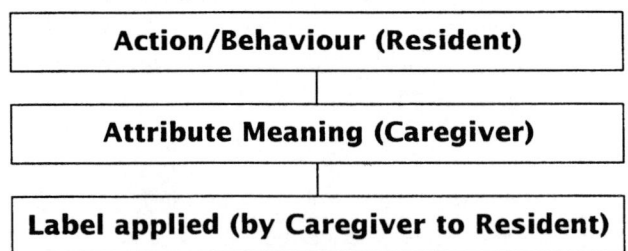

Figure 1

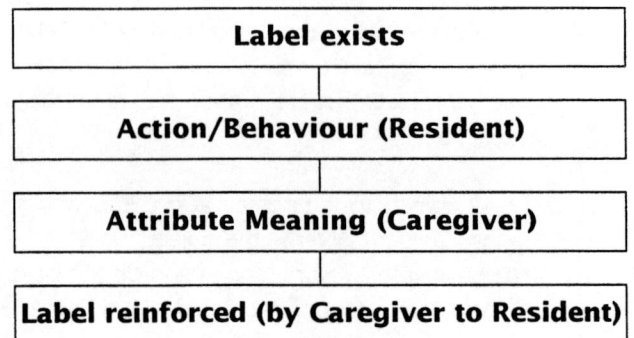

Figure 2

dering' behaviour (which is sometimes viewed as difficult) and outlines several types of 'wandering' that a person can engage in. These might be: an abnormal amount of time spent walking; an abnormal speed of walking; a repetitive pattern of walking round a set route; attempts to leave a building or room; or frequent occurrences of being brought back. In order to define what exactly the behaviour is it is therefore necessary to determine what are the words, gestures or actions and what is their frequency, duration, and quality.

The term behaviour therapy assumes that maladaptive behaviour is learned as a way of coping with stress, and techniques can be used to substitute new and more appropriate responses for maladaptive ones. A classic behavioural approach would consider what happened before the behaviour, the behaviour itself, and the consequences that may positively or negatively reinforce the behaviour. The theory is that the behaviour is being learned as a response to stimuli either directly before, or immediately after the behaviour has occurred. The behavioural approach would be to alter the experience surrounding the behaviour and therefore to change the behaviour. To use this approach, information would be systematically gathered about the circumstances surrounding the previously defined behaviour and a pattern would be sought that could then be interrupted by changing those circumstances. The system for gathering the behaviour might take the form of a chart (Fig.3).

However this type of approach tends to focus on the behaviour itself. A more person-centred approach would consider all factors affecting an individual's thought processes and feelings. The range of emotional responses that a person may have to their perceived circumstances will depend on past experiences and personality type. One person who has been outgoing and sociable and has travelled extensively is likely to be more self-confident than someone who has always kept to him or herself and has never left their home town.

Therefore if both of these people were to find themselves in a strange environment, which they are unable to make sense of because neurological impairment is causing them to be disorientated, one person would possibly feel at ease and the other would feel insecure. The shy person who is feeling insecure may express this by weeping, wandering, or withdrawing and becoming socially isolated. This person is less likely to demand answers by repetitive questions. This comparison of personality traits and past experiences demonstrates how important it is to know the personal context of an individual if the behaviour is to be understood.

Understanding the behaviour

A model for understanding the whole person, and all the factors that have an impact on behaviour, was developed and published by the University of Stirling (Burton, Chapman and Myers – fig 4). It seeks to lead caregivers to consider the personal context of the individual with dementia in terms of their past experiences and personality and also in the present context of the disability and ability of the person. It is also proposed that the degree of insight that a person has may affect the consequent emotional wellbeing, as a person will attribute a sense of failure or shame to their lowered level of ability. The thoughts and feelings of the person are recognised as being critical to the 'what happened before' stage of the behaviour episode. If this is recognised and sensitive caregiving can enable the person to think or feel more positively about their situation at that moment, the resulting behaviour will be much more positive.

Of equal importance is the caregiver's behaviour, which can be part of what happened before or the consequence, and can serve to support or undermine the person. This model recognises that the factors affecting the caregiver's behaviour are as complex as those affecting the person with dementia. In terms of the

Figure 3: Behaviour Chart

Name:					
Behaviour being monitored:					
Date	Time	Antecedent	Behaviour	Consequence	Person involved

caregiver's personal context, the skills base achieved through training is only one factor. Many care service providers assume that training alone will solve the problem. But the values and beliefs of the caregiver and the particular belief about the individual with dementia are often too deep for a 'quick fix' training course to address. Therefore serious attention must be given to finding out the values and beliefs of caregivers before recruiting to caring roles. The care service providers must also recognise the effect of the work environment on the caregivers. Are there rigid routines or heavy workloads that put pressure on the caregiver? Do colleagues put pressure on each other to ease the workload? Are there any pressures from outside of work that the caregiver is unable to leave behind and is bringing to the situation?

Finally the building itself may be contributing to the behaviour; it is important to consider the design and decor (see chapters 11-16). An unfamiliar building will cause anxiety and unease, too little stimuli will cause boredom and unrest, too much stimuli will cause distress and agitation. Careful observation of a person with dementia may reveal that a certain behaviour always occurs in the same environment and some adjustment of the features may resolve the problem.

Meeting the need

The purpose of applying a model like this is to remove the barriers that are causing the person to have an unmet need. It would be wonderful if we could solve every problem by adjusting the environment and our response, thus anticipating and meeting unmet need so that the behaviour would not be necessary. However, this is rather a naive expectation. It is likely that the many and varied personalities and experiences of those

for whom we care and those who provide the care will inevitably give rise to occasions when behaviours are misunderstood and help is needed to resolve the resulting conflicts.

A truly person-centred approach must also consider the medical disability of the individual, and not focus only on the social disability caused by expectations and interactions from others. It may be that neurological impairment is having a direct impact on a person's behaviour as a chemical imbalance occurs. For example, damage to the frontal lobe of the brain may lead to an inability to control emotional behaviour and lead to emotional outbursts or sexual disinhibition. If adapting the physical and the social environment does not reduce the behaviour, and the person is in a state of ill-being during these episodes then appropriate medication may offer some relief. Medication should never be used as a first resort or to provide relief to those around the person who is exhibiting the behaviour, but it does have a place in improving the quality of experience of the person with dementia. The use of medication as a means of managing and controlling behaviour is never to be condoned, but a person with dementia has as much right as any other to be offered medication that can offer relief from distress.

A situation may arise where the person with dementia is carrying out behaviours that those around him or her find unacceptable or distressing, but he or she is not in a state of illbeing. In this case it may be appropriate to consider helping the person move to live somewhere that is more accepting of that behaviour.

There are no simple solutions, but the challenge is to recognise the opportunity for giving support, for forging closer relationships, and for learning more about individuals. Therefore there are no challenging behaviours – just behaviours that give us opportunity for growth.

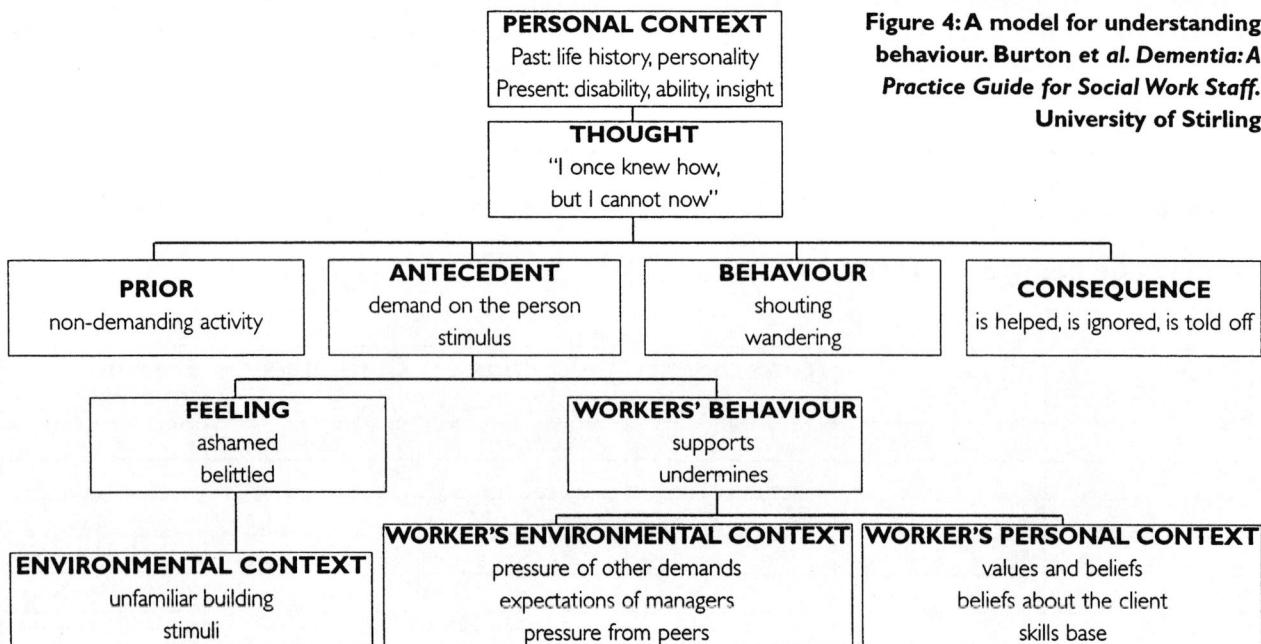

PERSONAL CONTEXT
Past: life history, personality
Present: disability, ability, insight

Figure 4: A model for understanding behaviour. Burton et al. Dementia: A Practice Guide for Social Work Staff. University of Stirling

THOUGHT
"I once knew how, but I cannot now"

PRIOR non-demanding activity	**ANTECEDENT** demand on the person stimulus	**BEHAVIOUR** shouting wandering	**CONSEQUENCE** is helped, is ignored, is told off

FEELING
ashamed
belittled

WORKERS' BEHAVIOUR
supports
undermines

ENVIRONMENTAL CONTEXT
unfamiliar building
stimuli

WORKER'S ENVIRONMENTAL CONTEXT
pressure of other demands
expectations of managers
pressure from peers

WORKER'S PERSONAL CONTEXT
values and beliefs
beliefs about the client
skills base

CHAPTER
SEVEN

A sudden change of need: nursing reassessment with the older person with dementia

JAN DEWING

Senior fellow in dementia care, Royal College of Nursing

*T*his chapter will consider what a sudden deterioration might mean for an older person and what nursing reassessment in such a situation should be concerned with. The issue of assessment and in particular nursing assessment of older people should not be considered in isolation from what is happening within the wider health and social care policy arena. Currently, there is a wave of policy activity surrounding older people including those living in long term care. For example: The Royal Commission on Long Term Care (1999) legislation on Care Standards and the proposed National Required Minimum Care Standards (Department of Health 1999)all of which will impact on older people living in long term care settings.

Central to much past and current policy activity are issues around what is said to be nursing and what is said to be personal care. The RCN believes that older people are entitled to free nursing care wherever they are nursed. An older person in a nursing home is there because they primarily require nursing. Central to understanding what comprises nursing, when it is needed, what is needed and how it is delivered is the activity of assessment and reassessment as carried out by registered nurses. The act of assessment and reassessment, because it is carried out by a registered nurse, helps to define what nursing care is and is not.

A sudden deterioration?

A sudden deterioration can be a change in a person's medical or health status that takes place instantaneously or over a very short period of time. Or it could be that the change has taken place over a longer period of time but is suddenly noticed by others. The change can bring with it a set of needs both for medical treatment and for nursing care. Understanding the implications of a sudden change in the condition of an older person with dementia requires gerontological attributes comprising different types of knowledge and skill. These attributes can be summarised as being:
• **Holistic practice and holistic knowledge:** bringing together different types of knowledge about the older

patient or resident as a person (at more than a superficial level)

• **Saliency:** seeing the most important and relevant issues in the situation and the most appropriate ways of responding to them according to the wishes of the older person

• **Knowing the patient:** as a person, and their typical pattern of responses, in order to make a skilled judgement about the most appropriate response

• **Moral agency:** a concern for responding to the person, respecting their dignity, protecting their personhood in times of vulnerability, helping the person to feel safe, providing comfort and maintaining the integrity in the relationship with that person

• **Skilled know-how:** performing in a way that appears fluid and seamless and highly proficient. Actions of the nurse reflect attunement to the situation and are shaped by the older person's responses.

These attributes do not exist in a vacuum; they require the ability to reflect on the effectiveness of practice, authority in and accountability for practice, therapeutic interpersonal relationships with team members and older people and a practice environment that enables a person-centred approach to the organisation of care services.

How and when a change or a sudden deterioration in a person is noticed can depend on the nurse, his or her values and beliefs about dementia, attitudes towards those with dementia, clinical skills and the relationship between nurse and older person. For example if the nurse believes it is usual for older people with dementia to rock themselves backwards and forwards (it is not) then they may not see this behaviour as a possible sign of psychological ill-being, physical discomfort or pain (Marzinski 1991; Hurley *et al* 1992).

Before a nurse even begins to reassess an older person's nursing needs he/she must have knowledge about the presentation of disease in early and later life and know that presentation can be very different. Signs and symptoms taken for granted in younger adults, the usual case studies referred to in most nursing texts, can be minimal or absent in older people (Heath and Schofield 1999). For example, left sided chest pain and shock in an acute heart attack may not be present. It may be replaced with a generalised feeling of being unwell. High temperatures with an infection are often reduced in older people thus masking the severity of the infection. Nurses working with older people need to know about ageing and how deterioration influences disease and illnesses. This knowledge is essential foundation for the development of holistic knowledge – such a vital part of assessment and reassessment.

A sudden change in an older person's health status will usually relate to one of the following areas:
• Mental confusion (increased or decreased activity; noisy or quiet)
• Falls or immobility
• Incontinence.

This alone is not always helpful as it is in the context of knowing the person that any changes in health status or behaviours begin to make sense. Putting these signs into context they might look something like the following:

Mr Patel doesn't seem easy to wake up. He usually wakes quite early, calling out for his wife, but this morning he is sleeping more deeply. He looks hot and sweaty. When he is rousable he is more confused than usual.

Miss Weston has been in the home for about one month. One afternoon she is found in the lounge looking very dazed and is disorientated, by her standards.

Len has got out of bed, unusually it's wet and he is acting in a very confused manner. At breakfast time he seems unable to eat his food and is spilling it on the table.

Kirsten seems unable to stand or walk. This has been the case for the last two days.

Mary, who is usually wandering actively around all day is sitting in a chair with her head in her hands making whimpering noises.

These changes are not experienced by the nurse as something dramatic and may not immediately seem life threatening, but they are sudden in terms of the older person's life span – a threat to their abilities, independence and quality of life.

Causes of deterioration

Older people with dementia may have other diseases and changes associated with ageing which affect them physically or mentally. Having dementia does not mean that diabetes, arthritis, changes in hearing and eyesight for example, will be absent. However, the older person with dementia may have little reserve to cope with physiological changes to their body. After all they are fighting minute to minute and day to day against changes to their self identity and personhood heaped onto them by the dementia process and, perhaps, an unhelpful psychosocial environment (Cheston and Bender 1999, Dewing 1999, Kitwood 1997).

Older people in general have a reduced reserve for fighting against disease and illness (Schofield 1999) but older people with dementia may be even more sensitive to changes in their state of health, even very small ones. For example, a lack of sleep or tiredness, medications given at the wrong time or additional medications given can cause a dramatic change in functional ability and cognitive abilities (Hopker 1999). Constipation is, of course well known for contributing to ill health and a change in an older person's cognitive and functional abilities (Rush and Schofield 1999).

Deterioration is multi-faceted. There can be a multitude of causes from discomfort and pain, the environment, sensory impairment, alcohol, physical illness, treatments especially drugs, psychological factors (Byrne and Arie 1990). There can also be a multitude of ways in which the older person with dementia demonstrates and experiences the effects of a sudden deterioration in their medical or health status.

Terminal deterioration

It is probably useful to consider for a moment that there are some people with advanced dementia in whom it is not possible to know what is going on. Any assessment is a challenging process as usually they cannot communicate their needs and seem to be unresponsive to care and the environment. Nursing reassessment with these older people must focus on the essentials of care, that is preserving dignity, respect for personhood, attention to nutrition and hydration and promotion of comfort and release from pain.

There are some older people who seem to deteriorate for no apparent reason. Certainly no medical causes can be found. How nurses choose to identify and work with this situation depends again on their knowledge base and experience but also on their own beliefs about life and death. Older people, including those with dementia, can sometimes seem able to control their dying and actively let go of their life. This is a fundamental issue that deserves a respectful and dignified response from nurses and family carers. Whatever events unfold, an older person must be re-assessed keeping central what is known about the person, the best course of action for that older person decided upon and a care plan developed and implemented by a registered nurse. There must be documented evidence to show these processes have taken place and that the whole team has been involved in the process.

Deterioration in older people with dementia

Changes in function and deterioration are more or less expected with dementia and often attributed simply to the dementia without further investigation (see Lovestone 1999). Nurses must question this assumption if they are to practise in a person-centred way. This culture leads to under-observation and under-reporting of changes in a person's health status. It is the school of thought that says everything that happens to a person with dementia is a result of the dementia (because it's a global cognitive condition). It is then just a short step to saying it doesn't really matter what is done or not done as the dementia means good health and rehabilitation are meaningless. This mind set highlights Tom Kitwood's fundamental principle that *the person* is what matters foremost and not the dementia (Kitwood 1997). This is not to say that dementia and its possible effects should be ignored. However, we are currently attributing too much to dementia. Applying the *person first* principle in situations where there is a sudden deterioration, therefore means looking at and beyond dementia for a reason to explain what is happening, doing what you know that person would want for themselves and not just what the nurse feels is the right thing to do. This can take experience, confidence and guts – in other words, an expert gerontological nurse with the attributes described earlier.

Nursing skills in reassessment

Nurses, support workers and family carers can notice quite subtle changes in residents. Often they are communicated in vague ways such as "She's just not right", "He's not his usual self today" or "She's off her food". Rather than shrugging this off the professional should tune in to hunches or gut instincts, ask more questions, look closely at the older person to see exactly what it is that's not right and also to try and find out what it is that's causing the change. It may then be possible to take action. However, it may be that the causes are ageing related and cannot be stopped. It will thus be most important to find out what difference the changes are making to the person's abilities and quality of life in order that compensatory actions can be taken.

Nurses and other professionals have a role in developing a positive culture of care, including the way the team works, that makes it acceptable for carers and support workers to voice their observations and concerns knowing that they will be listened to and acted on. As previously demonstrated, nurses clearly need to have a knowledge of the many diseases of ageing and how they affect older people, especially when they co-exist with dementia. However, it is the relationship these have with the person and how the person's potential for health is affected, not just how the diseases interact with each other, that is the central concern for nurses.

Nursing reassessment

Reassessment may need to take place in several phases. Initially, there may be life saving actions or actions that minimise serious complications for the older person's life or health. This involves assessment by the nurse and often takes place 'on the hoof' as decisions and actions can happen quickly. It may only be recorded as an event and the assessment part not captured. If this happens, apart from the various professional and legal implications of not keeping full records, valuable learning material for other members of the team to access has been lost. It is helpful to regard writing about care as an activity that promotes learning as well as providing evidence of accountability. Writing down any care records and sig-

nificant events enables reflection to take place. This is a useful learning opportunity both for an individual nurse but also for a team. Recording of the events surrounding a significant event such as when a person collapses or becomes unconscious is not all there is to nursing reassessment where there is a sudden deterioration.

Once the older person is stable a full and formal nursing reassessment is needed. The nursing reassessment is what happens once the significant event has been responded to. It is the consequences or change in ability (McCormack 1998) arising from a change in health status or a medical condition and how this is going to affect the older person with dementia that leads to a nursing reassessment of the older person's needs and abilities.

Before beginning any reassessment the nurse should ask herself:
• Why am I doing this re assessment?
• What is the aim of the re assessment?
• When should I reassess?
• How should I best obtain the information I need?
• How should I judge what this information means?
• How might the person function under different circumstances? (Barker 1997)

Skilled nursing assessment depends upon a variety of factors including: choosing the right time and place, the nurse being in the best mind set, knowing what information is important and how it will be used in care planning, having skills with interpreting information, selecting the right or best assessment tools and scales, good interpersonal and communication skills, identifying and building upon the older person's needs, strengths and assets rather than inabilities and dependencies (RCN 1998). Care plans that include statements such as "Mr Patel is unable to wash himself" or "Miss Weston can't feed herself" focus on inabilities and are generally the result of an assessment that has not been person-centred or built on ability or need. Those with statements such as "Len needs feeding" are only slightly better but are still nursing task focused and not person centred.

The RCN Assessment Tool (RCN 1997), will support nurses in undertaking a person centred assessment that focuses on abilities and strengths. The RCN Assessment Tool for Older People enables:
• Assessment of the older person's health status within categories of ability /need
• An assessment of stability and predictability giving a trigger for potential registered nurse input
• The identification of the need for registered nursing and non registered nursing input
• An estimate of the level and frequency of nursing intervention needed through four types of intervention (management, supervision, actual and directive care giving)
• An estimate of the number of registered nurse hours required
• The identification of evidence to support decision making and practice.

The RCN Assessment Tool offers a framework for assessment that includes activities of daily living familiar to most nurses, but they are linked to a comprehensive review of biography, health status, medical diagnosis personal circumstances, care needs and self care deficits. It is the reviewing all of these that enables a nursing care plan to be devised that is person-centred, focusing on abilities/need rather than task centred and depersonalised.

Summary

Reassessment is something that often happens informally on a day-to-day basis and it is good practice that this occurs. But where there has been a significant event or change in an older person's health status, abilities or needs, a detailed, recorded nursing reassessment is called for.

Reassessment of nursing need is a key nursing activity because it will detail the type and level of nursing intervention an older person requires. Nurses therefore have a responsibility to ensure they are knowledgeable and skilled in gerontological assessment. Structured reassessment through use of *The RCN Assessment Tool for Older People* offers nurses and older people with dementia living in homes a means of carrying out reassessment that is both person focused and builds on the person's remaining abilities and strengths. Use of the RCN tool also provides additional positive outcomes that are useful to the team and the organisation.

References

Barker P (1997) *Assessment in Psychiatric and Mental Health Nursing: In Search of the Whole Person.* Stanley Thomas, London.

Byrne E J and Arie T (1990) Coping with dementia in the elderly. In: Lawson DH (ed) *Current medicine 1*. Churchill Livingstone, Edinburgh.

Cheston R and Bender M (1999) *Understanding Dementia: The Man with the Worried Eyes.* Jessica Kingsley, London.

Department of Health (1999) *Fit For the Future? National Required Minimum Care Standards.* Department of Health, London.

Dewing J (1999) *When Your Heart wants to Remember: Person Centred Dementia Care.* RCN Continuing Professional Practice Update Unit 98. RCN, London.

Heath H and Schofield I eds (1999). *Healthy Ageing: Nursing Older People.* Mosby, London.

Hopker S (1999) *Drug treatments and Dementia.* Bradford Good Practice Guides. Jessica Kingsley, London.

Hurley AC Volicer BJ Hanrahan PA Houde S Volicer L (1992) Assessment of discomfort in advanced Alzheimer's patients. *Research in Nursing and Health* 15 369-377

Kitwood T (1997) *Dementia Reconsidered; The Person Comes First.* Open University Press, Buckingham.

Lovestone S (1999) Activities of daily living. In: McKeith G M Cummings JL Lovestone S Harvey RJ and Wilkinson D G (eds) *Outcome Measures in Alzheimer's Disease.* Dunitz, London.

Manley K and McCormack B (1997) *Exploring Expert Practice, Distance Learning Module, Msc in Nursing.* London, RCN.

Marzinski LR (1991) The tragedy of dementia: clinically assessing pain in the confused, non verbal elderly. *Journal of Gerontological Nursing* 17 25

McCormack, B. (1998) Maximising life potential. *Elderly Care* Vol. 10 (3) pp 42-43

RCN (1998) *What A Difference a Nurse Makes.* RCN , London.

RCN (1997) *RCN Assesment Tool for Older People.* RCN, London.

RCN (1997) *Guidelines for Assessing Mental Health Needs in Old Age.* RCN, London.

Royal Commission on Long Term Care (1999) *With Respect to Old Age: Long Term Care – Rights and Responsibilities.* Stationary Office, London.

Rush S and Schofield I (1999). Biological Support Needs In: Heath H and Schofield I eds (1999). *Healthy Ageing: Nursing Older People.* Mosby, London.

Schofield I (1999) Age related changes. In: Health H, Schofield I (eds) *Healthy Ageing: Nursing Older People.* Mosby, London.

CHAPTER EIGHT | The use and misuse of drugs in dementia

STEVE HOPKER

Consultant psychiatrist, Bradford

*I*n this paper I outline some of the pitfalls in overemphasising the medical framework when approaching people who are affected by dementia and refer to the benefits of employing a person-centred approach when considering drug treatments. I discuss the variety of problems affecting people in which drug treatments might be helpful, and provide an overview of the main groups of drugs that might be given (major and minor tranquillisers, antidepressants and 'antidementia' drugs), with reference to evidence about their therapeutic and adverse effects. I conclude with comments regarding future research needs.

Pitfalls of a dominant medical framework

Although (most) people affected by dementia have abnormal changes in their brains, an overly medical approach can lead to the domination of disease and disability when considering care and treatment. Thus, the person may viewed as an object, a case, whose behaviour is seen only in terms of brain pathology. As a result of this professionals may not relate to them empathically, as a fellow human being, but rather deal with them objectively and at a distance.

From this viewpoint it is natural to assume that they, and indeed their carers, are unable to make much objective and therefore valid comment upon their care, which must be organised for them by experts, especially those who know about brain disease, namely doctors.

This is of course a caricature of doctor-patient and doctor-carer relationships; most practitioners are aware of such problems and seek to combat them. Yet I suspect there will be resonances for those who have been involved with the care of persons with dementia, and perhaps other health problems. The point here is that although drug treatments are clearly a medical issue, they also may be drawn into the processes described above, much to the detriment of truly helpful care.

Many readers of this paper will be familiar with the notion of person centred care, championed by, among other people, the late Professor Tom Kitwood, who has been highly influential in my thinking about this topic. For those not familiar with this concept or his work, I would recommend in particular his book *Dementia*

Reconsidered: The person comes first (Kitwood 1997).

None of this in any way denies the reality of brain pathology or the value of technical expertise: rather, this approach suggests that brain pathology is but one aspect which should not unduly dominate care planning or, perhaps most crucially, set the cultural tone for interacting with the affected person and their family.

On the assumption that medical input is made in a balanced way, doctors can contribute to assessing:
- the presence and impact of physical illness
- therapeutic and adverse effects of current medication
- diagnostic status, eg of dementia syndromes and any other mental health problems
- types and degrees of risk.

Most significantly for this paper but also perhaps for those affected by dementia, doctors have a key role in reviewing and amending current medication and in prescribing new drug treatments.

What kinds of problems might be helped by drugs?

There are perhaps two key themes in the kinds of problems that people with dementia can face: first, their variety and second, their variability over time. This means that assessment must be holistic and continual.

As I have suggested, serious problems can arise directly from the way others relate to the person affected. In this section I have provided a summary of the types and frequencies of problems felt or shown by the individual. This was originally published in a paper by Tariot (1996). The table below shows the median (middle value) and the range of frequencies reported in published papers: I have reordered the list, putting the most common problems first.

Problem	median	range
withdrawn/passive	61%	21-88%
agitation	44%	10-90%
appetite disturbance	34%	12.5-77%
delusions/other abnormal thoughts	33.5%	10-73%
anxiety	31.8%	0-50%
hallucinations	28%	21-49%
sleep disturbance	27%	0-47%
verbal aggression	24%	11-51%
misperceptions/illusions	23%	1-49%
disturbed mood (usually depressed)	19%	0-86%
physical aggression	14.3%	0-46%
resistive/uncooperative	14%	27-65%

Note the wide range of frequencies for most of these problems: this is probably due to the variety of care settings from which the reports were made. Nonetheless, it would seem that some problems – such as passivity – are somewhat more common than difficult or aggressive behaviour.

These problems are sometimes found to occur together in syndromes with similarities to mental disorders affecting people without dementia. For example, disturbed appetite and sleep, alongside withdrawal, might suggest depression. It can be difficult to interview people with impaired recent memory or language, but there are suggestions from research that depressive syndromes are often not recognised, especially in people with dementia. This means that interventions such as reviewing care approaches or antidepressants may not be thought of.

It is of course vital to consider the context of a persons' problems. For example, someone who is resistive or verbally aggressive while being quickly dressed might be much less so if given as much time as possible to dress themselves. Thus, a review of care approaches, carer support or even care setting may well be indicated, before medication is considered.

In the following sections, various classes of drugs are outlined, with summaries of their potential benefits and disadvantages.

Major tranquillisers

This group includes some of the most commonly prescribed drugs for people affected by dementia. Sometimes termed 'antipsychotics', these drugs were first used in asylums in the 1950s, given typically to people diagnosed with psychoses such as schizophrenia, but soon afterwards to people diagnosed with dementia. Sometimes they are used in people with dementia to treat psychotic symptoms such as delusions or hallucinations, but much of the literature relates to attempts to treat agitation or aggression – ie use as tranquillisers.

Some of the more commonly given major tranquillisers are listed below, along with commercial names that are sometimes more familiar and possible starting dose. Naturally, an individual's dose will need to be tailored to their situation, including likely problems with adverse effects.

Drug	trade names	possible starting dose
		(total daily dose, often divided)
thioridazine	Melleril	30mg
chlorpromazine	Largactil	30mg
haloperidol	Haldol, Serenace	1mg
sulpiride	Dolmatil	200mg

Evidence for benefits

Despite the wide use of such drugs, there is little good quality evidence for their value in people affected by dementia who have problems such as agitation or aggressiveness. There seems to be a large 'placebo effect', perhaps because the agitation/aggression was related to a transient situation such as a relationship problem or short-lived physical illness.

At best, there seems to be a net likelihood of about one in five people given such drugs actually benefiting, which, given their adverse effects, is not impressive. Indeed, a recent review of thioridazine, which is very often prescribed, suggested that there is no clear evidence of benefit and that if it was being introduced now, as a new drug, it might well fail to be approved by the regulatory bodies.

Adverse effects

There is a wide range of adverse effects, which also vary between sub-groups of major tranquillisers and to some extent individual drugs. Most, however, can cause problems such as parkinsonism (stiffness and shaking – in 75 per cent of recipients), prolonged abnormal movements (sometimes called tardive dyskinesia – in 25-50 per cent) as well as sedation, falls, increased confusion, blurred vision, constipation, urinary retention and a 'zombie' or depressed feeling. Tardive dyskinesia, which is often disfiguring and if severe can be disabling, has the additional risk of becoming a long term problem, even after the offending drug is stopped.

Given this combination of high rates of prescribing, poor efficacy and risk of side effects, one might expect these drugs to be somewhat controversial, and indeed this has been the case – at least in the United States. Concerns over excessive prescribing in US nursing homes led, in the 1980s, to legislation specifying when such drugs should and should not be used, and how often they should be reviewed.

There still may be situations in which judicious use may be of value (for example, where psychotic symptoms are causing distress), but clearly dosage must be cautious and kept under review.

There are some newer types of major tranquillisers, called 'atypical' antipsychotics. They fall into this category because they have a much lower risk of causing disorders of movement such as parkinsonism. However, they do have other side effects, which vary from drug to drug – and the extent of any value to people with dementia is not well established.

Minor tranquillisers

Most of these drugs are part of the benzodiazepine group, of which the most well known is probably diazepam. Introduced in the 1960s as a substitute for the more toxic barbiturates, it was suggested at first that they were a non-addictive substitute – but experience proved otherwise. They are sometimes used to treat agitation, insomnia or aggression in persons affected by dementia. On the next page are listed some of the more commonly prescribed minor tranquillisers.

Drug	trade name	possible initial daily dosage
diazepam	Valium	2-5mg
nitrazepam	Mogadon	5mg
temazepam	Normison	10mg
lorazepam	Ativan	0.5-1mg
oxazepam	Serenid	30mg

Evidence for benefits

There have been very few trials of these drugs at any degree of quality in persons affected by dementia. There is possibly some short lived benefit in agitation or insomnia, but these drugs tend to lose their effectiveness over time, as explained below.

Adverse effects

Most reviews, and all those in recent years, advise great caution in prescribing minor tranquillisers to persons with dementia. This is in part due to problems with sedation, increased confusion, unsteadiness and proneness to falls – which have parallels to problems with major tranquillisers. Minor tranquillisers suppress normal breathing, but overall they do not have the wider range of adverse effects described with major tranquillisers.

Unfortunately, if prescribed for more than a month or so, all minor tranquillisers are liable to induce tolerance (the same dose no longer has the same effect), withdrawal symptoms occur if the drug is reduced or stopped and dependency may result. Since the problems of a person affected by dementia may well persist beyond such a short period, these drugs should in most cases be used only as a stop gap measure.

Antidepressants

Widely prescribed for depressive syndromes in the general population, antidepressants are quite often prescribed to persons who are thought possibly to be affected by dementia and depression, or just the latter – since depression can resemble dementia in some people. They are also sometimes given as alternatives to major or minor tranquillisers in persons with aggressiveness or agitated behavioural problems.

It is beyond the scope of this paper to describe the various types of antidepressant, but some examples are given below:

Drug	trade name	initial daily dose
amitriptyline	Tryptizol, Lentizol	25mg (rising to 100mg plus)
imipramine	Tofranil	10-30mg (rising to 100mg+)
lofepramine	Gamanil	140mg
fluoxetine	Prozac	20mg
sertraline	Lustral	50mg
venlafaxine	Effexor	75mg

Evidence for benefits

There are some better quality trials of antidepressants in persons with depressive and dementia syndromes: these generally found a benefit, though with a wide variation of degree. The extent of benefit may be less marked than for persons who have depression without dementia. There is a possible benefit in using antidepressants to reducing aggressive or restless behaviour in persons affected by dementia, but formal trials have yet to confirm this.

Adverse effects

These vary quite markedly, though antidepressants in the same group are often similar in terms of side effects. Thus, older 'tricyclic' drugs, like amitriptyline or imipramine tend to cause sedation, dry mouth, constipation and blurred vision, among other problems. These side effects can be less troublesome if the drug is introduced at a low dose and gradually increased.

Drugs such as fluoxetine and paroxetine are members of the newer group of 'SSRIs' (selective serotonin reuptake inhibitors – a name describing their action on a chemical linked to depression called serotonin). These drugs may cause sedation, but are conversely prone to cause agitation or insomnia, along with tremor and sweating.

There is some evidence, at least for the tricylic group, of an increased risk of falls (and fractured femurs) similar to that related to major or minor tranquillisers.

Although antidepressants do have a potential for numerous adverse effects, there is evidence that these are not perhaps so serious as those for tranquillisers: there is no evidence for risks of addiction as is the case for minor tranquillisers, and a very low risk (though not zero) of movement disorders.

'Antidementia drugs' and cognitive enhancers

Currently, drugs of this type fall into two broad groups: those aiming to prop up failing brain functions (specifically, low levels of a chemical called acetylcholine which is linked to memory) and those which in some way or other is thought to slow some of the disease processes which are associated with dementia syndrome. The evidence for therapeutic and adverse effects of these drugs will be mentioned in each section.

Drugs in the first category are sometimes called acetylcholinesterase inhibitors, or cognitive enhancers, as they inhibit a natural chemical called acetylcholinesterase, which inactivates acetylcholine, and therefore may boost levels of that chemical. Tacrine (Cognex) was the first of these, and was marketed in various countries, but was only licensed in the UK more recently and is not marketed here. More recently, donepezil (Aricept) and rivastigmine (Exelon) have become available. Galantamine (Reminyl) has also recently been granted a European licence.

Evidence for benefits

Those trials which have been published of the two drugs currently marketed in the UK, donepezil and rivastigmine, appear to show a range of responses, with about a one in four or five chance of a person showing a significant degree of benefit. The results relating to Activities of Daily Living Skills and to Quality of Life do not seem to be so clear, although these areas, especially the latter, are hard to assess in a formal trial so as to yield useful numbers.

Adverse effects

These are generally related to the drug's action, namely the boosting of acetylcholine (which has a number of functions): they can include nausea, loss of appetite, diarrhoea and sweating. Rates of such problems seem to be fairly low, perhaps around 5-10 per cent and vary between drugs, with tacrine perhaps having higher rates. Unfortunately tacrine is prone to cause harmful changes in liver function and for this reason is not a likely treatment choice.

'Antidementia' drugs, which may possibly slow the destructive processes in dementia include aspirin (at low doses this can reduce problems with poor blood flow, and may at higher doses reduce damaging inflammation), hydergine, extract of ginkgo biloba and vitamin E.

The evidence for benefits for most of these drugs is not extensive and not striking, although low dose aspirin is of proven value in reducing the risk of strokes and is advisable in people affected by dementias relating to impaired blood circulation, and hydergine is possibly of very modest benefit.

Looking ahead: future research

The new antidementia drugs are the product of an intensive period of investment: how many more cognitive enhancers will be developed is not clear, but the research initiative is now moving towards more direct 'antidementia' treatments, such as possible 'vaccinations' and other drugs – some of which are used in other areas, such as hormones, which may slow the progression of brain disease.

On the other hand, there does not seem to be much likelihood of extensive research into older treatments directed at emotional or behavioural problems (such as tranquillisers), which is understandable from a commercial perspective but may mean the somewhat unsatisfactory lack of good evidence for the use of drugs – which will probably continue to be extensive.

Finally, returning to the notion of a person-centred approach, while there has been some support for research in this field, this, along with other non-drug interventions, remains an area both of great promise, yet also vulnerable to underinvestment.

References

Kitwood T (1997) *Dementia Reconsidered.* OU Press, Buckingham.
Tariot PN (1996) Treatment strategies for agitation and psychosis in dementia. *J Clin Psychiatry* 57 Suppl 14 21-9.

Further reading

Hopker S (1999) *Drug Treatments and Dementia.* Jessica Kingsley, London.

Editor's note

Since this paper was first given by Dr Hopker, the UK National Institute of Clinical Excellence (NICE) has reviewed the use of three currently licensed anti-dementia drugs, donepezil (Aricept), rivastigmine (Exelon) and galantamine (Reminyl). It has concluded that the drugs have value in a limited number of people and should therefore be available free of charge to NHS patients, following specialist assessment and recommendation. Such patients would, of course, include clients resident in care homes.

CHAPTER
NINE

Training to improve dementia care in care homes

BRENDA BOWE & BUZ LOVEDAY
Dementia Training and Consultancy Services

Care practice is not just about what we *do*; it's about how we *think* as well. Every part of the caregiving process will be heavily influenced by the attitudes and opinions of caregiving staff and their managers. Everyone involved in the care of people with dementia will have a set of beliefs and assumptions – even if these are not conscious – and ultimately the standard of care in any establishment will depend heavily on these. Consider whether you agree or disagree with each of the following statements (which can be used as triggers for discussion during training):

- 'Staff should try to prevent people with dementia from expressing angry feelings.'
- 'Staff should pay at least as much attention to the emotional needs of people with dementia as they do to their physical needs.'
- 'When a person with dementia is asking for their mother, who you know is dead, they should always be gently reminded of the death.'
- 'People with dementia should be given medication to control their behaviour if they are creating problems.'
- 'People with dementia should be involved, as far as possible, in the planning of their own care.'
- 'Staff should keep a professional barrier between themselves and the people with dementia they are caring for.'
- 'People with dementia should have the right to take some risks.'
- 'If staff are not getting their own needs met, they may not be able to meet the needs of the people with dementia they are caring for.'
- 'People with dementia should be prevented from expressing any sexual feelings.'
- 'Staff who work with people with dementia need a lot of support.'
- 'Until there is a cure for dementia, there is not much that can be done to help people who have it.'
- 'The same routine around personal hygiene should be in place for all people with dementia.'
- 'How a person is affected by dementia can depend on the way they are cared for.'

Having thought about these contrasting opinions (all of which are alive and well in the minds of assorted workers across the country!) consider whether your positive opinions are reflected in care practice at your residential home. Perhaps you have a role in making it happen. Everyone involved in the care of people with dementia, whatever their job, has some part to play in influencing the care that is received. There may well be barriers to be overcome. Maybe you can think of strategies for doing this.

What type of care would be delivered by a careworker who holds the opinions you disagree with? Negative opinions about people with dementia will produce poor care, which typically involves social, emotional and/or psychological abuse. Tom Kitwood (1997) identified 17 types of 'malignant social psychology', or commonly occurring care practices which undermine the well-being of people with dementia. These include people with dementia being:

- ignored (Amy is sitting alone in a lounge, calling 'Nurse, nurse'. A careworker walks straight past Amy to the tea trolley, and wheels it past Amy and out of the room, without so much as a 'hello')
- infantilised ('Daisy's lovely', says a worker, patting the 92-year-old Daisy on the head, 'but she can be very naughty')
- disempowered (Patrick is slowly buttoning up his cardigan when an impatient worker takes over and does it for him, saying 'Oh Patrick, all the buttons are in the wrong place')

When we realise the devastating effects practices such as these can have on people with dementia, we may well feel angry with those responsible for such abuses. But we cannot afford to blame individuals for poor care practice. Rather we should understand and attempt to address the causes of such negative attitudes and poor care:

- lack of information and understanding
- lack of insight
- lack of specific skills
- lack of motivation
- lack of direction
- lack of support from managers and organisation
- lack of resources.

In considering this list we need to look at responsibilities at all levels of an organisation. Training has a part to play in addressing these deficits, but it is only one out of a number of contributions. Training is only a temporary visitor. It can only achieve a lasting influence if it works in tandem with the organisation's philosophy, practice and resources. Equally vital are the local manager's style, attitudes, approach, role-modelling and commitment to ongoing improvements in the type and standard of care received by each individual. From chief executive to handyperson there needs to be a consistent reflection of person-centred values and practices.

So what is person-centred care? The term can be used very loosely. I would suggest that whatever interventions are used, care practice can only be person-centred if it is directed by the needs of the individual as a whole person, giving as much weight to emotional and psychological needs as to physical needs. Caregivers must work proactively to gather information about each individual's needs and their identity. They must also look for the ways that individuals make their needs known, often through their behaviour which should, therefore, never be viewed as meaningless. The process of care should be rooted in the belief that what we do makes a difference, both positively and negatively; the goal of care should be to help the person with dementia maintain or achieve a sense of well-being as their neurological impairment advances.

Person-centred care is based on an understanding of dementia as a disability. In any disability the person will be influenced by a number of factors in addition to the disability itself. Take John, for example – a man not with dementia but with a purely physical disability. He has been involved in a traffic accident and his spinal cord has been severed in the lumbar area. He is paralysed from the waist down and therefore completely unable to walk. Countless people with such a disability lead active, fulfilled lives and are able to live independently, to transport themselves and to work. However, in addition to his physical disability there are other factors in John's life which disable him further:

ENVIRONMENTAL FACTORS
• House of poor design for wheelchair
• Only two wide doors
• No ramp at front door
• No suitable transport
• No stairlift

SOCIAL PSYCHOLOGICAL FACTORS
• Partner and family can't cope and expect him to 'get on with it'
• Friends fuss over him
• Public treat him like a child

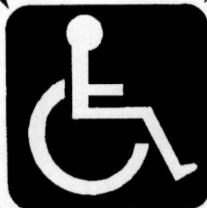

HEALTH PROBLEMS
• Poor eyesight
• Arthritis in neck and shoulders

PERSONALITY AND LIFE HISTORY
• Has always dealt well with life's knocks
• Good sense of humour
• Has had to give up a job which he loved

It is clear to see how John's disability is magnified by an environment which confines him, a social psychology which undermines him and health problems which hamper him further. His personality might just enable him to combat some of these other negative influences; on the other hand his coping strategies might be badly knocked and unable to help him this time. In many ways, the other factors are more disabling to John than his spinal injury.

Dementia is like this too: the person is disabled by their neurological impairment but other factors influence just how disabling this needs to be. If we replace John's disability with dementia, we can consider how environmental, social psychological, personality/life history and health factors could impact on the disability of dementia:

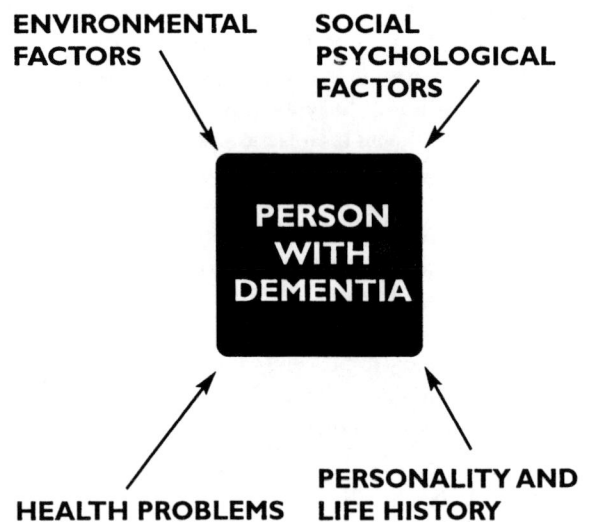

ENVIRONMENTAL FACTORS **SOCIAL PSYCHOLOGICAL FACTORS**

PERSON WITH DEMENTIA

HEALTH PROBLEMS **PERSONALITY AND LIFE HISTORY**

The environment plays a large role in assisting or disabling a person with dementia. Examples of factors which could have a negative influence include:
• Long corridors with unmarked doors (which could increase disorientation and render a person unable to find the toilet or their own room)
• Chairs which are too low or which otherwise restrict a person's freedom of movement (apparent incontinence could result from a person not being able to respond promptly to signals from their bladder)
• Dim lighting (which could increase perceptual difficulties and communication problems as well as making it even harder for a person with dementia to orientate themselves)
• Rooms which all look the same (so the person mistakenly walks into another resident's room and gets into their bed; the other resident wakes up with a justifiable terror that they are being attacked)
• A shortage of private space (which could easily result in an undermining of dignity, perhaps leading to withdrawal or an aggressive response)
• A lack of personal belongings (making it even harder for the person to feel grounded; increasing the sense of missing home).

Thus a person with minimal neurological impairment could become completely disorientated, incontinent, unable to recognise staff, withdrawn and constantly asking to go home – and all of this, simply through the effects of the environment. Most of these factors would be so easy to rectify. At the very least we should aim to provide an environment which does not make matters worse for people with dementia. And wherever possible the environment should be used positively to help compensate for a person's difficulties (for example, a picture of her beloved cat on Eileen's bedroom door ensures that she is always able to find her own room).

It is similarly important to make sure that social psychological factors are not increasing the person with dementia's level of disability. The examples of 'malignant social psychology' given earlier on in this chapter could easily result in the person with dementia being disempowered, losing self-care abilities and motivation, having to express their needs through challenging behaviour and becoming depressed. Health problems or any other disability or deficit which the person might have in addition to their neurological impairment can also increase the effects of their dementia. Consider how pain, for example, will often decrease a person's attention span and make thinking muddled and tempers frayed. Hearing difficulties or other sensory deficits can severely compound communication problems. It is essential to ensure that people with dementia are not being further disabled through physical problems which should be addressed.

And as for an individual's personality and life history... we may not be able to make any changes here, but getting to know an individual really well can help us find ways of counteracting any factors which are increasing their disability. Graham Stokes (Dementia Care '98 Conference) gave the example of an individual whose apparent incontinence on moving into a residential home was actually due to a lifelong hatred of public toilets; she could not bear to use the communal toilets on the ground floor of the residential home. If we understand how a person's own preferences and past experiences can influence their behaviour, we are enabled to think creatively about ways of working with this individual to minimise such difficulties.

If there is one basic message which any training programme needs to get across to caregiving staff it is the need to minimise any factors which are compounding the person's disability, especially any which they might be contributing themselves. Only then is it possible to work to enhance the person's quality of life. Training, therefore, needs to be an eye-opening experience for staff. It goes beyond simply teaching people to do something. Perhaps the kind of training we are referring to could, more accurately, be termed a process of personal and professional development. It needs to involve:

• Promoting appropriate attitudes: for example, care-workers' ways of looking at their clients' behaviour; their ways of developing relationships; their views and feelings about old age, neediness, difference. In some ways, the process of training and development needs to get at the very heart of what makes them who they are – their values, their beliefs, their moral code. Some people come into care work with appropriate attitudes already formed – if so, training has much to build on. But frequently we do need to work to try to change attitudes and we must recognise that this is a slow and complex – but entirely possible – process.
• Developing skills: the skills required for dementia care are many and specialised. At the forefront are complex interpersonal skills including highly developed non-verbal communication, active listening and even counselling, as well as skills in groupwork, time management, physical caregiving, etc.
• Enhancing knowledge: in order to give good care, it is necessary to understand something about the nature of dementia and especially to focus on the importance of gaining knowledge about each individual person with dementia.
• Encouraging reflection: through our experiences we learn, but only if we can clearly, critically and constructively reflect on these experiences. Reflection enables staff to learn from their own and their colleagues' successes and mistakes. Through this, understanding and self awareness can be sharpened.
• Lowering of defensive barriers: person centred care cannot exist where 'us and them' barriers loom large. Each of us have different defences, inhibitions, patterns of behaviour which can get in the way of forming close, personhood-maintaining relationships with those who have dementia. Training must address these defences.

The bottom line is that if staff are empowered to believe that what they do really makes a difference then there is much more motivation to make this difference a positive rather than a negative one. Perhaps negative attitudes and opinions can best be shifted if we become fully aware of just how much power and influence we, through these opinions, can have on the lives of people with dementia.

Reference
Kitwood T (1997) Dementia Reconsidered: The person comes first. Open University Press, Buckingham.

CHAPTER TEN | Staff roles in care homes: suit the word to the action

STEPHEN JUDD
Executive director, Hammond Care Group, Sydney, Australia

*W*e hear a lot about designing our residential facilities for people with dementia and the need for social environments which are not institutional but homely and domestic. We hear about the need to ensure that we encourage independence, autonomy and self-esteem rather than dependency.

But one of the great inhibitors in Australia to achieving these ideals has been the highly institutionalised work practices in residential aged care facilities which have been governed by the employment 'awards' – the terms and conditions agreed to by the industry associations and the relevant unions.

Until 1999 in New South Wales, Australia, the employment conditions for assisted living hostels were tightly constrained by the award. What a personal care assistant (PCA) could do and what a domestic staff member could do were clearly delineated. Domestics cleaned, cooked and laundered; PCAs attended to the personal care needs of the resident.

When the Hammond Care Group established The Meadows in 1995, we sought to establish a staffing model that more closely identified with the care ideals we were promoting. The Meadows comprises three separate cottages, each with 12-14 residents with dementia. Each cottage has its own kitchen, laundry, and backyard. Very few services are delivered into each cottage and we wanted to ensure that the number of faces seen by residents about the place was as small as possible.

We looked to have a staffing model that had two staff members dedicated to work within each cottage during the daytime shifts, with one staff member for all cottages through the night shift. The average number of hours per resident per week was more than 17. However, we wanted staff to enable residents to be as independent as possible: they could launder and put out the washing, vacuum the floor or sweep the path and cook in the kitchen. In short, residents performed activities of daily living as much as possible and in much the same way as they did before.

The relevant award struggled and groaned with such a model: it presumed a culture of dependency where "hotel" services were carried out by others: the food was cooked by others, the tables were set for others and the laundry was sent out. What we were looking for was an agreement with our staff where they were responsible for enabling residents to undertake activities of daily living as much as possible, supporting individual residents by compensating for personal dysfunction.

Enterprising solution

The solution was an Enterprise Agreement between staff and the organisation. That agreement would be the framework for the employment relationship between staff and employer. The first step towards an Enterprise Agreement (EA) was the establishment of a consultative committee, consisting of elected employee representatives, the manager of the facility and the human resources manager. The purpose of this committee was to shape the conditions of the EA.

From the perspective of Hammond, the primary interest was to have an employment relationship which reflected the style of care that we were seeking to promote. For the staff, the top priority was not money: a greater priority was to have a job title which more accurately reflected who they were, their expertise and their roles. Instead of the generic 'personal care assistant' they wanted to be known as 'specialist dementia carers'.

Hammond adopted a two-phase approach to the enterprise agreement. It is not a trivial matter to ask staff to leave the security of an industry-wide award which is negotiated and supported by the union. They must feel totally comfortable. So, in the first stage, the two parties sought to have an initial 12-month agreement. We used the award as a template from which we deleted clauses which were irrelevant to our situation, such as allowances for people who sleep over in a facility. Then we removed anomalies: we allowed staff to cash in twice each year what was known as 'counter leave', the loadings which accrued when working public holidays. But, most importantly, we also agreed upon job descriptions which accurately reflected what both staff and Hammond wanted achieved in these facilities.

Challenges

The Enterprise Agreement negotiations were not without challenges. As was required under state legislation, Hammond advised the relevant union when we commenced the EA process. There was no response. However, after both Hammond and the staff had concluded their negotiations, and both parties were about to take the EA to the Industrial Commission for ratification, the union challenged the fact that it had not been included in the bargaining process and that there was no substantial pay increase in the agreement.

Hammond had no problem with the union delegates attending meetings as observers but not as part of the consultative team. The staff agreed to this view: they knew they had access to the union for advice when they wanted it, but did not want the it to take over the process from them.

Eventually, staff voted overwhelmingly for the Enterprise Agreement in a secret ballot conducted by the Electoral Commission and the Industrial Commission ratified it.

The second stage took a lot longer than the first. We spent a lot of time unpacking the roles, developing competencies, and setting up a 360-degree appraisal system and more focused training programs. Hammond felt the total wage bill should remain the same but be better distributed by increasing the base rate and reducing the number of shift allowances and penalty rates. However, the staff as a whole did not agree. In the end, it was agreed that pay rates in the agreement would reflect those of the industrial award.

The major benefit for the organisation has not been financial but in having an employment agreement with staff that reflects its philosophy of care. It is interesting to note that, within 18 months of our first agreement with staff, the union agreed to changes to the industrial award that enabled far more flexibility. It is good that they have responded so positively to the EA that they initially opposed, and ensured greater flexibility for the industry as a whole.

However, the key element of the Enterprise Agreement has always been the organisational environment. As Hammond's human resource manager noted, 'There is no way that we would have got to first base with the agreement if the culture of the organisation had not been what it was. The employees are multi-skilled, flexible and customer-focused. And management leads by coaching rather than taking an I-tell, you-do approach.'

• This chapter first appeared as an article in the *Journal of Dementia Care* 8(1) 10.

Living and working together

CHAPTER ELEVEN

ALISON JOHNSON
Independent voluntary sector consultant

A **good home for people with dementia is one where residents, staff, relatives and members of the wider community together live life to the full in, as far as possible, exactly the same way that we all live out our normal lives. We must never lose sight of the fact that people with dementia are primarily people and that a good care home should primarily be a home. How can we then ensure that, in the words of Professor Faith Gibson, our residents continue to feel 'fully paid up members of the human race', coming to the beginning of each day with eager anticipation and to the end of the day with a sense of achievement and satisfaction?**

In an earlier presentation at a *Journal of Dementia Care* conference, I developed the idea that activities of daily living were equally as important to the maintenance of well-being as the more traditional activities programmes favoured in many care homes, where residents are expected to take part in bingo, carpet bowls and collage making. This view was shared by the author of a recent article in *Community Care* which looked at life in sheltered housing in Holland. He made this comment about the vibrant life he observed within the complex: 'It's not down to bingo and Christmas parties. Residents seemed livelier because there were *things to do as a matter of course*, rather than social events just added on.' (Benn 2000, my emphasis)

'Things to do as a matter of course.' This surely is the key to a fulfilling life in a care home for people with dementia. Activities don't have to be structured: they are not a means of passing time, or keeping residents occupied, they are the stuff of life itself. Activity means everything we do, because everything has the potential to be therapeutic. Our task is to provide opportunities for our residents to continue to live and work in such a way that their personhood is affirmed and they can feel fulfilled. In this way we will be able to care for them in a rounded and holistic way paying attention to their physical, mental, emotional and spiritual needs.

Activities are therefore too important to leave to one profession or one individual activities organiser. It must become the responsibility of every single member of the staff – and that includes those who clean or garden or cook meals. When I visited Australia on a study tour, I saw 'diversional therapists' who did run activities themselves but were seen primarily as facilitators rather than as people who 'took the residents off over there away from everything and kept them busy doing something'. They also had an important role in educating staff and providing guidance on how to incorporate activities into everyday life and care.

Life story

The place to begin in this approach to activities is where we must always begin – with the individual resident. To understand the needs of the person with dementia we must know as much as possible about his or her life and work. Was Mrs Jones a housewife or did she go out to work? Did Mr Briggs live in India at one stage of his life? What happened to Mr Brown in the war? Have we ever studied the framed certificate on Mr Anderson's wall? An attempt to find answers to these questions and to get to know as much as we can about every other aspect of our residents' lives will help us to understand the person now – especially as people with dementia are often living in an earlier period of their lives.

A good home will encourage residents and their families to develop a life story book which includes information, photographs and other memorabilia which help to capture memories. *A Pocket Book of Memories* has been developed for this purpose (Sheppard & Rusted 1999). Another idea developed by Faith in Elderly People Leeds is a memory box which contains meaningful memory joggers, personal items and photos. Both book and box can help provide answers to some of our questions about our residents, but are also invaluable for reflection on past times, for sharing with other residents or visitors and for using with new staff to introduce the residents to them. In addition our care plans should closely document likes and dislikes and personal preferences.

How then can we develop the life and work of our home to take account of the individual needs of our residents? It would of course be easier if there were enough staff or volunteers for one-to-one attention. Failing this, we need to look at the daily routine and see how residents could be involved in the various components of daily living – personal maintenance, work, recreation, physical activity, social interaction and spiritual development.

Personal maintenance

We begin with what Faith Gibson calls personal maintenance. An important aspect of life for us all is caring for oneself – getting washed and dressed, bathing, eating meals, washing our hair and so on. Staff members can brush a resident's hair roughly dragging out the tangles or can brush with care almost like a massage. Similarly smoothing hand cream into arthritic hands can be done in a perfunctory way or be a blessing to someone who misses the closeness of the affectionate touch of a caring relative.

Most of our residents will need help with bathing or showering. This activity helps to ensure personal hygiene, but for all of us a bath can be much more than simply a place to get clean. Staff can ensure that residents are given a choice of bath or shower, a choice of time of day and regularity and the privacy of a pleasant, warm and domestic-style bathroom.

The relaxation of a leisurely bath can be a balm for the soul and for a resident may be a peaceful oasis in a communal setting and an opportunity to share deeper conversation with a trusted member of the care staff. And afterwards the choice of clothes to wear, the rediscovery of forgotten garments and the opportunity of reminiscing about them make an everyday task a pleasurable activity.

Similarly we all have to eat and drink to ensure that we have sufficient nutrition and fluid to maintain life. But having a meal is so much more than eating or drinking. For older people with dementia who live in a care home, it can be a significant event in a day when not very much may be happening! Engaging in the familiar social ritual of a meal not only triggers past memory but provides a milepost in the day.

It is important again to ensure choice of menu, allowing for individual likes and dislikes (we don't lose these because we have dementia). We can still allow flexibility in timing and location – a late meal for a resident who has had a visitor or breakfast in bed for those who don't choose company early in the day. But think too of the nourishment of the spirit we all experience through sharing meals with friends, engaging in conversation or celebrating special occasions. Might it be possible from time to time to encourage staff and residents to share meals together and welcome families and friends from the community to eat in the dining room?

And what of the end of the day? Our bed is so much more than simply a place to get a good night's sleep ready for the next day. Many of us look forward to bedtime as an opportunity to unwind, relax, escape from our families, read, watch television, have an intimate conversation with a parent or spouse or a time to think or pray. What about some calming music or relaxing massage for a resident at bedtime? And does someone say 'goodnight and sleep well' to each resident?

Work

In the home

Having cared for our physical needs, most of us spend a large part of the day in productive activity, otherwise known as work. For many of our female residents, this activity was centred in the home. In the survey carried out by the Centre for Policy on Ageing as a part of the consultation for *Fit for the Future* (DoH 1999), a resident remarks: 'I like to help the staff around the place and wash up. I don't want to give up. I've always liked being busy.'

This comment applies equally to residents with dementia, many of whom believe that they still have household responsibilities. A continuing role with domestic tasks has numerous benefits for our residents – it builds confidence and self esteem, maintains skills, makes them feel useful and valued and provides continued social interaction – the opposite from the boredom, apathy and futility of life which so many people experience in care homes.

Many of us who have visited dementia care facilities in Australia have come back with enduring memories of homes where the kitchen was the centre of the life and work of the home. Often a part of the main lounge and dining area, it was accessible to residents who were able to help as much as they wished with, for example potato peeling, sandwich making or washing up. In the dining room residents laid the tables and cleared away afterwards. The smell of cooking permeated the home. Life seemed normal, the atmosphere peaceful and close relationships between staff and residents developed through shared activity.

There are many reasons why we may not feel able to replicate this here – for example staff roles, regulation and design. However Methodist Homes for one has attempted to do so by providing a kitchen as part of the lounge in its new dementia care homes.

At Mayfields, Ellesmere Port, which was recently commended by the Audit Commission, a group of residents regularly makes cakes. This involves much discussion and reminiscence about recipes, suitable ingredients and their packaging, types of scales and preferences for gas or electric cookers. The cake making itself brings back memories of the feel and the texture of the ingredients and the smell of the cakes cooking in the kitchen adjoining the lounge speaks of home. And what pleasure there is in having something to share with other residents and staff or to sell at the regular coffee morning.

Another area of the work of the home where residents may well like to be involved is in the laundry. Washing at least some of their clothes, pegging them out in the garden and folding aired garments and replacing them in drawers are all comforting tasks that remind residents of home, of normality and of continuing role, and give satisfaction in a task achieved. In Australia I saw a happy group polishing their cherished silver ornaments and reminiscing on their origin and meaning to them. Similarly many residents much prefer to dust their own rooms rather than have a domestic sweep in and carry out the task rapidly but without love and care.

Many of our residents spent a lifetime caring for children and husbands. In Australia I saw many examples of residents who believed they still had family responsibilities and who were comforted and affirmed by caring for a doll. Although some are concerned about infantilising and undermining the dignity of a resident who plays with a doll or teddy bear, others point to examples of adults with all their mental powers who take a bear to bed. We must never dismiss any activity out of hand without looking carefully at its benefits to the individual resident.

In the same way a resident who has always had a pet can find solace in the companionship of a toy dog. This can be a perfect companion, giving meaning and purpose to life and providing a topic of conversation with staff and visitors. If you've spent all your life caring for an animal, why must you stop when living in a care home?

Men also need opportunities to be involved in work around the home. These may be domestic tasks but for this generation of men it is more likely to be DIY or gardening. Every Australian man has his shed in the garden where he likes to potter and most homes included at least one. Several had chicken runs and most supplied an outside toilet too! Many residents were involved in gardening, including some who grew vegetables for the kitchen. At a day centre in Sydney the men with dementia daily swept up the leaves, just as they would have done at home. In Tasmania I saw a car in the grounds so that those who could no longer drive could continue to polish and care for a vehicle.

Outside the home

And what of those whose work took them outside the home? We often find residents are anxious to go out after breakfast and it is clear that for many this is linked with a feeling that there is work to be done. It is important therefore that we find out about the working lives of each individual resident and then seek to provide some sort of opportunity for continuing involvement in that sort of activity.

In a home south of Brisbane I saw a room set aside as an office for the use of residents. A desk was available with paper, pens, staplers, hole punches and all the other impedimenta which surround those who work in offices. A number of men and women used this office from time to time and felt at home and reassured by this familiar environment. In another home, an engineer tinkered happily in the courtyard with a large and greasy machine and in yet another I was told of a nursing sister who had always worked at night. She slept during the day and shared the life of the home at night with the night staff!

It is important that in these and all our work activities

we ensure that as far as possible residents will not experience failure. As well as helping to maintain cognitive and other skills such work must be achievable. Thus Mrs Howard may well still be able to wash her blouse by hand – but is unlikely to recall how to operate the washing machine. Mr Brown can remember how to plant leeks but may not be able to start the motor mower or be safe operating it.

Thus, engaging in familiar work activity, even if sometimes simulated, can allow a resident a sense of continuing value, purpose and fulfilment – which no amount of sitting around or playing carpet bowls can achieve.

Recreation

Nevertheless life is of course more than work, and we all need recreation. Often this is the only activity found in a care home. But we most enjoy relaxation when we have chosen it or when we find time to relax after our work. The Rev Fred Pratt Green, a former resident at the Methodist home in Norwich, captured this most tellingly in a poem about life in a care home which concludes:

Doing nothing, I observe,
is only boring
when there is nothing to do.

Today I want to do nothing
because of things
I am supposed to want to do.

Our residents need to have the choice of taking part in activities or declining to do so and opting to watch or to retire to their rooms. Table games, arts and crafts, quizzes and puzzles can all be enjoyed by people with dementia and we must never underestimate latent abilities, or the possibility of learning new activities in old age. A woman who has never sewn in her life is now at the age of 84 finding enormous pleasure in making a cross-stitch hassock for the parish church. A carer tells of how her Mum who never used to sing now sings often and with gusto. Another resident rediscovered the pleasure of knitting with the patient assistance of a friend.

We can often stimulate memory by showing videos of old films, looking at old magazines, reading aloud or reciting poetry. Often if we begin a poem, old song or nursery rhyme, the pattern and orderly sequence of sounds enables someone else to continue right to the end. I was greatly moved when visiting a home in Toowoomba to meet an elderly woman who was able to say little but who, in response to my request, played *Waltzing Matilda* on the piano. In another home, a lady sung beautifully to the pleasure of her friends. Those of us with a faith can bear witness to the joy of residents, sometimes with severe dementia, who are nevertheless able to join in the Lord's Prayer or the 23rd Psalm. Such skills and memories are there dormant in so many residents, if only we can find the key to unlock them.

Recreation can of course also be passive rather than active but is nevertheless an important part of life. A specialist multi-sensory room is a bonus. Equipped with soft textures, gently moving light, relaxed sound, warmth and pleasant smells it can be a joy to residents and staff alike. But there are numerous other ways that residents can enjoy relaxation through the use of massage and aromatherapy as part of the getting up or going to bed routine and light and music and other forms of sensory stimulation can be provided in any lounge or resident's room. Such stimuli often seem to bypass the blocks to communication which have developed in the brain.

Physical activity

Physical activity is also a very important part of life. Although people with dementia may lack the memory or drive to exercise we can still make opportunities for this during the day. For the more fit there may be continued delight in walking in the garden or to the shops, preferably with the companionship of a valued member of staff. Some may still be able to swim. For others physical activity may be confined to a slow walk to the dining room on the arm of a member of staff. Don't be tempted to use a wheelchair for the sake of speed.

Keep-fit is not just an important way of mobilising arthritic joints and improving overall fitness but can provide a wonderful combination of music and movement and refreshment for both body and spirit. Singing along with the familiar tunes and the general fun and banter that goes with exercise can often make this activity a highlight of the week – and can be easily adapted for those who need to remain seated. Many people with dementia are agitated or wander, and these energies can often be effectively channelled into exercise of some sort.

Social interaction

We have already several times touched on a vital further area of important activity for all human beings. This is the basic need for continuing social interaction. We have seen how mealtimes are an opportunity for this, we have looked at working together in the home through shared domestic activity, we have seen how much better a walk can be enjoyed when accompanied by a friend or member of staff and what pleasure can be gained from a shared keep fit session.

So often in the past, people with dementia were dehumanised and staff believed that they were an empty shell without need for social interaction. People with dementia lived together in a home but in the deepest sense were profoundly alone. Those who carry out Dementia Care Mapping often discover very little social interaction for those with dementia who are quiet and cause no trouble.

How then can social interaction be encouraged in a care home? Staff often feel that they must always be 'doing things for' residents rather than 'being with' them. But often the two activities can be combined. How about a care assistant ironing while talking to a resident? Or having a chat or laugh while washing up or folding laundry?

Each resident needs to feel part of the community and to experience tenderness, closeness and the soothing of pain and distress. The reassurance of attachments to care staff or to other residents will help them to function well, to feel part of the shared life of a group and to enjoy activities through which they can continue to express themselves.

However, staff need also to be clear that just being with a resident is an activity in itself. Residents in care homes frequently complain that the staff don't have time to talk. And staff have the same complaint. An experienced social worker is quoted as saying: 'There's just no time any more for the job to be meaningful and I miss that.'

She had no time to sit and be, sit and talk, with the people she was in contact with day to day.

Staff need the ability to listen, accept and understand. An Australian nursing home manager writes of the happy relationship she nurtures between staff and residents where: 'It is great to see nurses sit and chat with the group without feeling pushed to be busy bees. A discussion about local events or a child's illness or a recipe can go on for 20 minutes. The staff member has to be prepared to "waste the time".'

An unachievable dream or an important contribution to a positive and caring environment?

Spiritual development

And finally what of the spiritual development of people with dementia? We must be clear that spirituality transcends the purely religious and can be discerned in moments of awe and wonder, in experiences of life which transport one beyond the mundane and in relationships with others that give meaning and purpose to life. For many, but certainly not for all, this spirituality may come from a relationship with God but we must never believe that those without adherence to a particular faith do not have spiritual needs or are not spiritually aware.

We have already identified ways in which, through relationships and social interaction in the home, we can respond to this spiritual dimension of life. We have also looked at how a doll or soft toy can bring comfort and a sense of being needed. In many homes, the presence of a dog or cat, a fish tank or aviary can give enormous pleasure. A pet offers constant interest and stimulus – stroking and patting it and talking to it and about it with other residents and visitors. The Pat-a-Dog scheme will supply visiting dogs for homes unable to cope with their own, and sometimes a staff member is delighted to bring his or her own dog to work.

We need only look outside the window to nurture a continuing sense of wonder in our residents. I still remember the Australian home in Queensland where residents and staff were closely observing a bird which had nested in the courtyard and was raising her family there. The bird family had even become a regular part of the daily record. We can all share the beauty of a rainbow or frost on the trees, the swelling buds in spring or the colour of the autumn leaves.

In conclusion, every small, intentional act of kindness can be seen as an activity and should be valued as such. We must never dismiss anything we do with residents as pointless because our residents will forget. People with dementia will recall the emotion of joy, respect, wonder or security even if they cannot remember what they have been doing or why.

If we are able through our life and work in the community we call home to draw together enough joyful and meaningful activities and interactions, our residents with dementia will come to the end of the day with the feeling of satisfaction and well-being which is the right of every person.

References and further reading

Bell V (1997) Carer support is cost-effective. *Journal of Dementia Care* 5(6) 11.

Benn M (2000) Talking a good game. *Community Care* 19 March 14.

Broughton M & Johnson A (1998) Activity and community involvement. In *The care assistant's guide to working with people with dementia.* Hawker Publications, London.

Department of Health (1999) *Fit for the Future* (Department of Health).

Garratt S ed (1995) *Rethinking Dementia.* Melbourne Ausmed Publications, Australia.

Pratt Green F (1991) *The Last Lap.* Stainer and Bell.

Johnson A (1998) All play and no work. *Journal of Dementia Care* 6(6) 25-27.

Sheppard L & Rusted J (1999) *A Pocket Book of Memories.* Hawker Publications, London.

Marshall M (1996) *I can't place this place at all.* Venture Press.

Phillips M (2000) Let's go Dutch. *Community Care* 10 Feb 26.

CHAPTER TWELVE | Sharing activities: a way to bring back the pleasure of caring

CAROLE ARCHIBALD

Senior fieldworker at the Dementia Services Development Centre, University of Stirling. Illustrations by Anne Rodgers.*

I have long been convinced of the massive potential of activities in helping people with dementia, easing their disability and making life more pleasurable (Archibald 1990 & 1993). The use of activities is part of what has become everyday vocabulary in dementia work – a person-centred approach to care (Kitwood 1994).

What I have found, however, is that sometimes person-centred care can have a narrow focus, including only the person with dementia. My intention here is not to minimise this approach, which has been a huge step forward. However if we think that dementia is a disability which affects all the family and indeed the staff who are involved, then I would argue that a person-centred approach needs to be applied to all concerned.

I would like here to explore ways in which family carers might be helped to be involved in activities, if that is their wish, and how this might benefit both the person with dementia and also staff. In compiling our latest activities publication (Archibald & Murphy 1999) we surveyed the literature, consulted with family carers, professional carers, including staff working in long-term care services, domiciliary and day care services, and volunteers – all of which reinforced our view that involving family carers in enjoyable activities could have many benefits.

An easy option?

Involving family carers is not necessarily an easy option. As many staff would acknowledge, the issue is surrounded by complexities and difficulties – but there are also many rewards. What we have found is that success involves work and commitment by all parties. It involves some letting go of power by staff. It involves an acceptance that happy families can and do exist, but also accepting the complex nature of some family relationships which mean they might not want to be involved. Staff need to have some knowledge about activities; not simply the kinds of activities available, though that is important, but also the reasons why we do activities and how they can be used strategically to involve family carers and benefit people with dementia.

As professionals we have a knowledge about dementia based on caring for a number of people, sometimes

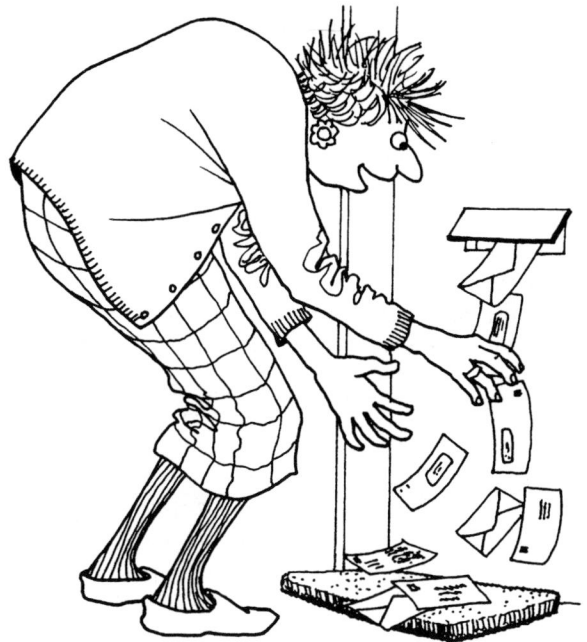

based on many years' experience. This can be shared with family carers. What I would suggest here is that we could do more to tap into the unique knowledge that family carers have of the person they are caring for and importantly, look at ways that this knowledge can be taken note of, acted on, and given the status it deserves.

Life story work (Murphy 1994) has to be the first step. Readers might see this as hardly a revolutionary suggestion. Life story work is now a commonplace activity, but my impression talking to staff and visiting services is that there are many ways this information, and the activity of information gathering, might be used more creatively. For example, how we can use the carer's special knowledge of the person with dementia to help to us to know, and indeed find the essence of the person so that we can use this information to provide relevant activities. This might include how family carers can use both the compilation of, and the life history book itself as an activity. The following case study illustrates how the compilation of a life story book helped one family. (All the case studies are taken from Archibald & Murphy 1999).

Elsie and Martha

Elsie had a diagnosis of dementia and lived in a nursing home. Her daughter Martha taught in the local secondary school and had three teenage children at home; she visited Elsie three times a week.

When Martha came to the nursing home she was tired, felt guilty and didn't know what to do and say to her mother during visits. She had never really had a close relationship with her mother. To fill the time during visiting she brought in food to give her mother. This was a source of real annoyance to staff because Elsie would then refuse her evening meal. Martha would talk to other visiting carers, check her mother's clothes, then leave.

Increasingly the visits were a burden and Martha wondered how much longer she could go on. She decided to speak to her mother's key worker, gradually grew to trust her and spoke in depth about her feelings, and lack of feelings, for her mother. She was able to talk about the difficulties she experienced at visiting times, when she felt at a loss to know what to do with her mother – realising that she had never really known her.

The key worker suggested the first step might be for them both to think about compiling a life story book for Elsie. This would help both Martha and the key worker to get to know Elsie better. The process was started after permission was sought from and granted by Elsie.

Compiling a life story book has many potential benefits: enabling the key worker to plan care centred around Elsie's needs based on her past and present life, so that she can appreciate Elsie as a person; and helping Martha to get to know her mother in some depth before it is too late. It could provide her with an opportunity to 'work' with her mother when she came to visit; and it could bring a degree of intimacy which she had never experienced with her mother.

Martha was asked to bring a whole lot of (old and new) photographs to the home. This request needed to be repeated twice as Martha was busy and the process entailed going through her mother's possessions, which she was reluctant to do. The key worker again stressed that the life history book was a store for Elsie's (failing) memory, and reminded her how much all the people involved would benefit.

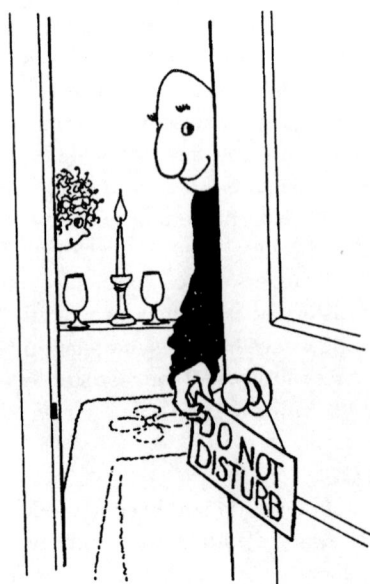

Martha did at last, with the aid of her own daughter and over a series of visits, bring in a pile of photos. Together she and her mother, and sometimes Martha's daughter, sorted out the photos Elsie wanted in her book. In large clear writing her grand daughter then wrote a short summary under each photo, using Elsie's own words. From this exercise staff learned a great deal about Elsie. For example, she had worked in London during the war, sleeping many nights in the underground. Although witness to the awful destruction during the Blitz, she looked back to this time as one of her 'finest hours'. She became animated when speaking about this time, and loved Vera Lynn songs. A whole range of activities stemmed from this discovery, and for Martha visits often became a pleasure.

The pleasure component is very important. Family carers are often too tired, after basic care-giving tasks or other commitments, to even think about activities. (There are parallels here with professional carers, particularly those working in long-term care services). This needs to be acknowledged. By using activities, giving carers a range of enjoyable activity ideas, we can help bring back the pleasure component to caring – even when the person is dying, as this next case study illustrates.

Jane and Pat

Jane had became very frail over the five years that she had had dementia. Her daughter Pat, with whom she lived, was aware that her mum would probably not be around next year. As it was autumn, Pat decided she would plant some bulbs to be ready for Christmas. She spread the kitchen table with newspapers, brought some bulb compost, and with her mother sitting watching she planted the bulbs. Pat asked her mother to firm down the compost around the bulbs, and with help her mother did so. The bulbs were watered and placed in a dark cupboard, to be brought out when they started to grow and establish a root system. When they had finished, Pat and her mother had a cup of tea and a cake. Jane seemed calm and peaceful, sitting quietly while Pat tidied up.

By Christmas Jane was terminally ill in bed. Pat and the district nurse worked together to care for Jane at home. Using aromatherapy oils Pat gave her mother gentle hand and face massage. She also played pieces of music which she knew were Jane's favourites. A lovely ambience was created, peaceful and caring. Sitting unobtrusively on the window sill, the pink, mauve and white hyacinths planted in the autumn perfumed the room, testimony to the activity they shared.

Betty and John

Betty and John had been married for over 50 years. Betty had dementia and because of increasing difficulties she had been admitted to a nursing home. They were a devoted couple and John visited the nursing home once or twice a day. John built up a trusting relationship with Betty's key worker and revealed to her that he missed the physical aspects of his relationship with Betty as much as the social aspects. The key worker explored with John what things they did together before her admission. John reported that he gave Betty her bath, he massaged her feet as she really liked this, and he slept with her.

Some delicate work with staff was required here; they initially felt uncomfortable with John providing intimate care for his wife, and also with the idea of sleeping in the same bedroom. It might help with his needs, but what about Betty, staff asked. The care plan decided on was that Betty would have a bath twice a week, unless she needed one more often, and John would help with this. He would massage Betty's feet not just at bath times but on other visits, and he could do this in Betty's room. There was not enough room for a double bed in Betty's small bedroom but there was room for a bed chair. It was therefore decided by everyone that once a week Betty and John could have a meal together in Betty's room, and John could stay the night.

These interventions were monitored to gauge the effects on Betty in terms of well-being. She showed no signs of ill-being and positively enjoyed the foot massage. The plan worked well for John. He became active in the carers group in the home. He was also able, as time went on, to spend less time in the home – once a day rather than twice a day – and to regain contact with some of his bowling club friends.

Activities and challenging behaviour

Activities can be employed strategically with carers to help with challenging situations. Using a problem solving approach the following case study illustrates how this might be achieved.

Muriel and Peter

Muriel lived with her husband Peter. She had previously worked as a lawyer's secretary and had been very efficient and well liked in her job. She was forced to retire early because of developing memory problems and was subsequently diagnosed as having dementia. At home, Muriel kept losing many letters including the electricity bills, and became angry and abusive to her husband when he asked where she had put them.

When asked to map when Muriel picked up the letters, Peter noted it was first thing in the morning when the post arrived, although she sometimes started to pick up letters in the afternoon. What happened before the picking up of the letters was that Muriel had her breakfast, and then had a shower and got dressed. Her husband then started to do the dishes and tidy the house leaving Muriel sitting and (her husband conceded) bored. The mail arrived and Muriel started to open it and then 'put it away' with any other letters lying around, if Peter did not keep watch. After she had put the letters away she appeared happy for a time – if Peter did not ask her where she had put the letters.

Looking at Muriel's life story, understanding that part of her work for many years was to attend to the mail and process it in the morning, it was decided that this knowledge could be usefully deployed. A mini office was set up for Muriel in the dining room, with 'mail' and files for her to sort it into. This occupied Muriel happily for half an hour, which enabled her husband to clear up the kitchen. He then brought her a cup of coffee for her 'coffee break' which was much appreciated, before she went with him to do the shopping. In the afternoon he asked if she would help him sort the mail and again, using this activity strategically, he was able to prepare the meal while Muriel was happily and productively engaged.

This activity helped for only three months, but essentially what her husband had learned was the problem solving process. With help, he was able to apply it to other difficult situations. He was in effect able to achieve a sense of mastery over the situation, as was Muriel.

Sharing ideas

Many family carers in their own homes provide a range of ideas when caring for their person with dementia. We need to explore these ideas and perhaps at carer groups share them with other carers (as some already do). What we can do is provide carers with further ideas – a repertoire in which they can engage, based on the needs of the person with dementia and, indeed, their own needs. Whether the person with dementia is living in the community or in long term care, involving carers in activities, if that is their wish, has many benefits that repay the increase in energy involved.

References

Archibald C (1990) *Activities*. Dementia Services Development Centre, Stirling.

Archibald C (1993) *Activities 2*. Dementia Services Development Centre, Stirling.

Archibald C, Murphy C (eds) (1999) *Activities and People with Dementia: involving family carers*. Dementia Services Development Centre, Stirling.

Kitwood T, Bredin K (1994) *Person to Person: A Guide to Care of those with failing Mental Powers* (2nd edition). Gale Centre Publications, Essex.

Murphy C (1994) *"It started with a seashell" Life story work and people with dementia*. Dementia Services Development Centre, Stirling.

*Illustrations are taken from Archibald & Murphy (1999).

• This chapter first appeared as an article in the *Journal of Dementia Care* 7(4) 20-22.

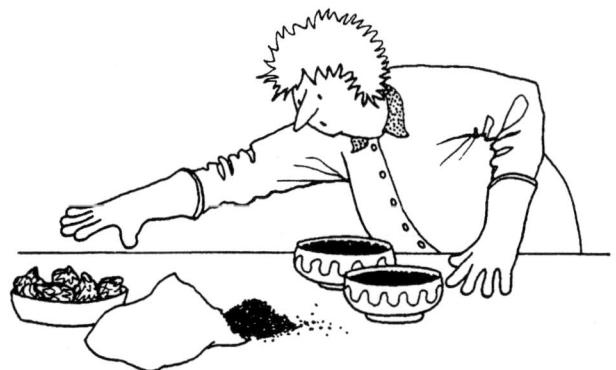

Environment and activity: a sea change at Kirklands

CHAPTER THIRTEEN

ANTHEA INNES
Researcher, Bradford Dementia Group

Kirklands residential home in Cumbria volunteered to participate in a Bradford Dementia Group/Anchor Trust collaborative research project. In working with the staff and residents there, I have been impressed by how much staff have done, in a very short period of time, to improve the care they provide for people with dementia.

Part of the project involved all staff participating in an education programme spanning four months. During this time staff began to act on their learning and implement several ideas they had discussed in training sessions.

One of the first things staff began to do was spend more time with their residents talking and utilizing forms of non-verbal communication. They began to develop the life history work they had made a tentative start on and ultimately produced life history material on all residents, much of this very detailed and artistically presented.

The topic of the environment caught staff interest and immediate plans were made and acted upon. The home was due for redecoration and staff made use of this opportunity to decorate the home, taking into account the ideas of the residents' group and the writings of people like Mary Marshall on the environment.

Frames around toilet doors on both floors and all wings of the home were painted the same colour to encourage and enable residents to locate toilets in any part of the building (a number of residents at Kirklands are very mobile and will walk to all parts of the home). The management at Kirklands wish to move away from institutionalized care and accordingly did not lock cupboard doors; this led to residents removing objects and many items becoming misplaced. Cupboard doors were thus painted the same colour as the walls to avoid attention being drawn to these doors. Each wing of the home was painted in a slightly different colour to enable residents to distinguish between them.

This has been taken a step further with the staff team which predominantly works in a given wing, putting enormous effort in to the "theming" of each wing. This process built on the information the team had gained about residents during life history work. Thus one wing has become a music and dance wing – one resident had been a dance teacher, another two used to be dancers and another had particularly enjoyed playing the piano and singing. Another wing has taken on the theme of the sea as this had been a popular holiday destination for several residents and the home is close to a seaside resort. One of the home's assistant managers made use of the chance encounter she had with a pub manager during a lunch break on a training course in Leeds. The pub had a sea theme and was about to change this and all the props were sold very cheaply, including an anchor – the name of the voluntary organisation Kirklands is part of. If residents want to handle or take away any items from these displays, staff are happy with that.

Another wing has taken advantage of the lake location and murals depicting local beauty spots have led to further reminiscing about past outings. Overall, the theming of corridors has led to much discussion, the prime reason for the initiative, and helped residents to find their rooms easily – an extra bonus.

The bathroom was pretty dismal and during training sessions staff discussed in depth how it could be made more welcoming – it was where they often spent a lot of good one-to-one time with residents. After discussion and a look at the budget, a local artist was commissioned to come in and design a wall mural that would take into account the client group.

A mural to remember

Residents have picked up on many aspects of this mural – a bright and amusing seaside scene with beach huts, bathers, a donkey ride and fairground. For one resident, the image of the donkey leads to discussion and her singing the Christmas carol Little Donkey. Others talk about their time at the sea, others comment on the facial expressions of the characters and begin to reminisce about people they knew/know who look like that.

Life history work reinforced staff perceptions that animals were important to their client group (and one wing has taken on a Cumbrian wildlife theme). The home had a dog which had recently died and staff were reluctant to replace it quickly; they overcame their own reservations when they realized how important the new dog was to residents.

The dog was introduced to one man with whom staff often found it difficult to work; it received a warm welcome and now sleeps in his room sometimes, alleviating problems staff had previously when the resident attempted to pull them into his bed. Rabbits were also purchased to give residents who liked to stroke the dog for long periods of time (which the dog didn't always appreciate) the opportunity to touch and stroke an animal content to sleep on their laps.

The staff at Kirklands are hugely committed to the care of all residents within the home and have instigated many fundraising initiatives to fund their endeavours. The home is based in a tight-knit community which has been generous in its contributions.

Many people have attempted to improve the environment of their care setting. What has impressed me so much at Kirklands are the achievements in a short time span and the huge motivation of staff – a great example of what a lot can be achieved in a short time.

• This chapter first appeared as an article in the *Journal of Dementia Care* 7(6) 23.

Environment and activity: reminiscence by recreation

CHAPTER FOURTEEN

MARY MᶜILWAINE & JOHN KILLICK
Mary McIlwaine, care assistant in a dementia care home in Belfast, talks to John Killick.

*I*t all began with my mother. In 1984 she began asking what day it was – over and over again – and not getting washed, wearing her shoes on the wrong feet and not cleaning her house. To be honest, we were ashamed of her. We thought at first she was just seeking attention from us.

She had 11 children. My sister and I were the youngest, and she was very close to us. Even though we were married ourselves and had our own families, we never left her out. When we went on family holidays we took it in turns to bring her along with us. She had had a hard time bringing us up: I remember when she did without food to give it to us. She never complained, was always cheerful, never letting us see when she was unhappy.

But 1984 changed our lives – her strange behaviour really got us down. When we eventually sent for the doctor he diagnosed dementia and told us that it would get worse. It was a lot easier when we understood what was behind the way she acted. Pity overcame our sense of frustration. Our love grew stronger, and the protection we gave her was the same gift she had given us.

At this point in time my only frustration was how I was going to find ways of helping her to pass the long day. Then I bought tapes of the old songs that Mum had sung herself when we were children. She remembered them and was able to sing all the words. Yet at the same time she was unable to hold a conversation with us. Our love and the music contented her.

Encounters with loneliness

I decided to apply for a care assistant post advertised in the local paper. I thought maybe by helping other old people I could learn new ways of helping Mum. The job was visiting old people who lived on their own. The first day out in the community meeting my clients I was shocked: it was all the loneliness, the fear, the neglect that I encountered. By the time that first day was over I decided that I would help all these people, and my mother would be my teacher.

I realised at this stage that activities like "reminiscence" were very important. Each day I visited someone who was confused I tried to gather another few pieces for the jigsaw that I was putting together. I was gradually building up a series of pictures of their lives, what they best liked doing in their pasts. One lady talked a lot about a bird she had had as a child so I bought her one, along with a secondhand birdcage. This made her very happy.

A gentleman who had suffered a severe stroke had been looked after by his wife for years. I went in regularly to give her a break. He was no longer able to hold a conversation or move. We were very quickly thoroughly bored with each other. Then I thought of the game of Ludo. It wasn't too complicated and anyone could play it. I found out that this had been a favourite activity of the couple before the dementia had struck. After a few months the man was throwing the dice by himself, and was deeply satisfied by this simple act. His wife said that I had achieved more for him than the physiotherapist had done.

Concentrating on the past

After a year of this work I was asked to go and work in what they called an 'EMI unit'. I had only been used to one-to-one working, so the day I started there I was distressed when I looked at the residents. They reminded me of mice in a cage, aimlessly going round and round. I took one lady by the hand and led her into the sitting room. Four or five others followed, and soon we were all enjoying a sing-song; I had learned the words and music from my mother's tapes.

I decided to concentrate on the past and went around secondhand shops where I bought a tin bath and a washboard. I placed them on a chair in the sittingroom, filled the basin with water, and left a towel and a bar of soap beside them. Within a short space of time I saw residents rolling up their sleeves and walking to the bath where they got stuck into the washing without any prompting.

Now I work in Shankill House, a residential home on the Shankill Road in Belfast. I have tried to put into practice here all the things I have learned from my previous experiences.

I asked my officer-in-charge for the use of a room which I converted to an old-style kitchen. I went to the shops again and bought old furniture, a gas light and other bits and pieces. Over the years I have kept on adding items and many have been donated. I have made the room as realistic as possible, and find that when I walk into it with residents I am really privileged to be walking into their pasts with them. The quality of memories from individuals who are really very confused is remarkable.

My next project was to provide somewhere special for the men (though I have found that some of the ladies really appreciate it too!). That is a bar, modelled on one of yesteryear, with appropriate posters round the walls. I've found furniture, bottles and beermats that fit with the period. Once a week or more I spend part of an evening with five or six gentlemen residents, listening, while they reminisce over pints of Guinness. And the craic* is good, I can tell you.

Many of our residents worked in the mills, which were a staple industry in these parts. So I also collect yarn and pieces of linen. I have a work pass that was issued for the men during the War. We decided that it wasn't sufficient to talk about these experiences: we should try acting them too. On St Patrick's Day many of the residents, some of their relatives and I improvised a play based on their stories of hard times. People took the parts of the hard-pressed wife, the drunken husband, the granny; some of it was sombre, and some of it brought hearty laughter. Drama is an activity I should very much like to develop.

Digging for memories

I also regard the garden as a very important agent of reminiscence. It isn't just somewhere to relax. Residents can employ four of their five senses (and if tea is served, all of them!). From the frailest to the fittest, everyone can draw benefit from this resource. It stimulates recall of outdoor experiences, and we have enhanced this by pro-viding examples of garden and street furniture. Apart from benches we have old streetlamps, a postbox, bicycles and mangles. Fitter residents can help with the upkeep of the flowerbeds. A garden, I find, is one of the pleasantest places in which to reminisce.

I am sometimes asked whether the elderly people with whom I work talk much about 'The Troubles'. The answer is very little. Sometimes the subject surfaces as funny stories, but people seldom refer to the terrifying experiences they have had. I think the reason for this must be that we have lived through what we refer to as 'The Riots' all our lives. Some of our oldest residents even remember the violent times which began in 1912. For most of us it is a part of our normal everyday existence; we have been conditioned to a state of war.

I always had a fear of school, and many elderly people in our society, whose education was very strict and narrow, feel the same. So I avoid any formal reminiscence sessions about that part of their lives.

Also, I avoid asking direct questions like 'Did you have money?' because I know some did and some did not but everyone has their pride. Instead, I use drama. In character I'd say, 'I pawned the lad's shoes.' This brings people out and in no time they're saying, 'Many's the time I went to the pawn.'

The secret is, I have found, to make finding out about the past a pleasurable activity. I'm doing it all the time but I never once use the term "reminiscence".

*Craic = lively social atmosphere and conversation.

• This chapter first appeared as an article in the *Journal of Dementia Care* 7(6) 24-25.

CHAPTER FIFTEEN | Environment: how it helps to see dementia as a disability

MARY MARSHALL

Director of the Dementia Services Development Centre,
University of Stirling

*T*he built environment can have a fundamental effect on a person with dementia: probably greater than on people who are mentally fit.

As far as design is concerned it is helpful to see dementia as a disability. This approach provides clear pointers to the disabilities for which a building needs to compensate. Dementia as a disability is characterised by:

• impaired memory
• impaired reasoning
• impaired ability to learn
• high level of stress
• acute sensitivity to the social
and the built environment.

The broad design implications of this are – or should be – obvious, at the general level. Buildings should not rely on the person having any memory of where they are or how they got there. Buildings should not rely on people remembering where to go. Buildings should minimise stress.

Design for Dementia (1998)* describes 18 buildings which I and the other editors consider achieve this effectively. We believe that the expertise should be made easily available to all concerned, and hope that as they are brought together in this book, readers will see design features as a whole. Introductory chapters draw out some of the lessons to be learned.

Disease or disability?

It can be helpful to differentiate between a disease model and a disability model in approaching design for dementia, since the majority of current buildings are based on the former. They should not be seen as mutually exclusive but rather as having a difference in emphasis. The disease model exemplifies definitions of dementia such as:

Dementia is a group of progressive diseases of the brain that slowly affect all the functions of the mind and lead to a deterioration in a person's ability to concentrate, remember and reason. It can affect every area of human thinking, feeling and reasoning. (Murphy 1990)

This approach to dementia care would tend to focus on

the inevitability of decline. Design considerations would be to keep people comfortable, safe and clean and to provide a building which takes account of behaviour such as wandering. In other words this approach does not prioritise the potential for buildings to assist functioning and prevent behaviour difficulties.

This approach is still the one held by the majority of professionals in the field of dementia care, although the disability approach seems to be more widely accepted in Australia. The disease approach still therefore imbues the design briefs written for architects and, since it is the view held by most of the public, it is the one shared by most architects too. It tends to result in large, clinical units. If the potential for therapeutic design is embraced at all by people adopting a disease model, it tends to be in designing buildings for those in the early stages of dementia.

Of course not all health services are unaware of the impact of design on people with dementia, nor are non-medical models always better. In our experience some of the most sensitive design features can be in medical and nursing settings whereas there are some very disabling buildings provided by welfare agencies.

International consensus

Design for people with dementia has not been subjected to the scrutiny of research in the same way as, for example, medication has. Work on the impact of specific aspects of design is very rare.

Given the paucity of research, it is significant however that there is an almost unanimous consensus about good design for dementia. Certain buildings have had a major impact, in part because of their energetic proponents. The CADE units of New South Wales, Australia and the Corinne Dolan Alzheimer Centre, Heather Hill, Chardon, Ohio, are widely quoted as exemplars. There are two ways of summarising this international consensus. One is the agreement on principles, the other the agreement on design features.

The consensus on principles of design includes:
• design should compensate for disability
• design should maximise independence
• design should enhance self-esteem and confidence
• design should demonstrate care for staff
• design should be orientating and understandable
• design should reinforce personal identity
• design should welcome relatives and the local community
• design should allow control of stimuli.

The consensus on design features includes:

- small size
- familiar, domestic, homely in style
- plenty of scope for ordinary activities (unit kitchens, washing lines, garden sheds)
- unobtrusive concern for safety
- different rooms for different functions
- age-appropriate furniture and fittings
- safe outside space
- single rooms big enough for lots of personal belongings
- good signage and multiple cues where possible eg sight, smell, sound
- use of objects rather than colour for orientation
- enhancement of visual access
- controlled stimuli, especially noise.

The selection of buildings

The buildings in this book meet these criteria to a notable extent and have an additional ingredient – they are pleasing buildings in themselves. In other words, good design for people with dementia has to have the same qualities that any good building has. We are not suggesting that buildings for people with dementia can be built to a formula. Architects need to take the brief to meet the criteria and then create a pleasing place to live.

Unresolved issues

There are a great range of issues which make designing for dementia a challenge even with a high degree of international consensus on the desired outcome. These include:

Cost

Cost is the most often quoted reason for not providing therapeutic design. There are numerous aspects to this. Here I will mention only a couple. The first is the issue of size. Small scale is at the top of the list of key design features. What this actually means is widely divergent. The *gruppeboendes* (group living flats) in Sweden house between six and eight people. The Scottish health service guidelines have consistently recommended eight or ten. Heather Hill in Ohio has 12 people in each unit. The maximum size of any unit in this book is 14 in the actual living unit (although the overall numbers in any cluster of units may be greater).

This is a cost issue, primarily because of the staffing implications. Staff is the major cost (or expense) consideration. The usual aim is to provide the minimum number of staff for a group of people with dementia to achieve good care. Excluding cooks and domestic staff and including activity staff this is usually 1:4-1:7; although it depends greatly on the needs of the people being cared for. Providing units in multiples of 4-7 is usually seen as the only cost-effective way to proceed. Many units deliberately not included in the book house

20 people with five staff, which is plainly indivisible except into units of six, which are not perceived as practical.

The second cost issue we wish to mention is that of designing for groups with different needs. People with dementia are far from a homogenous group, not least in the extent of their concomitant physical disabilities which, along with behaviour, is the way usually used to differentiate groups.

There are design implications for both issues. People with 'challenging' behaviours, for example, may need a great deal more visual access in the sense that they need to be able to see the staff and the staff need to be able to see them. It is clearly cheapest to build a standard building – which is how the larger nursing home companies achieve savings. However, this will not work with dementia care.

Regulations

Every county has fire and environmental health regulations which are essential to ensure that people using buildings which are not their homes are not put at risk. Fire regulations are usually concerned with ensuring that people can get out of a building or into a fire protected space with all speed. They usually specify the distance between any one safe area and the next, and are particularly concerned with rooms in which fire risks are greatest, such as kitchens and boiler rooms.

Environmental health regulations are concerned with transmission of disease through contaminated surfaces related to food preparation and consumption.

There are numerous difficulties with this apparently sensible system of legislation and inspection. The first is the tension which exists about the nature of the buildings in which people with dementia live when they are unable to live at home. They are classed as institutions or public buildings which are subject to very stringent regulation. The aim of most of the design principles and features listed above is that the person with dementia is living in a group environment as much like a normal house as possible.

The provision of a normal kitchen with normal fittings is, for example, an essential component of such an approach. Yet this is rarely acceptable to fire officers. If they agree at all it is only with stern requirements for a fireproof room which means that the kitchen is either sealed off and unrecognisable, or the unit is divided by fireproof walls in such a way that concepts of domesticity and orientation are severely compromised.

A normal kitchen is often unacceptable to environmental health officers too who require stainless steel and coolers in a kitchen. They often also require the installation of a small additional sink for handwashing, which is thoroughly confusing for people with dementia.

This seems to be a particularly British problem. In Australia the requirements for a small shared dwelling are less institutional and more flexible.

Since Aldersgate Village, South Australia opened in 1984 there has been greater recognition that these dwellings are houses, not institutions. In Sweden the principles of domestic design for people with dementia override the usual regulations. Indeed the regulations specify the characteristics of dementia design.

It also seems that British regulations have not kept pace with technological changes such as effective sprinkler systems, smoke alarms and the trend towards providing a safe space, rather than evacuation, when dealing with mentally or physically disabled people.

Another difficulty is the interpretation of the legislation which varies greatly over the UK. Some officers are much more cautious than others. It is an expensive and often delaying business to take issue with each interpretation.

Cultural appropriateness

If we genuinely believe that people with dementia retain their past memories longer than their present, we should provide designs which make sense in an era or a style familiar to the residents as younger people. There are several challenges to this:

One is that the units have a mixed population in terms of class, ethnic background, occupational history. A homogenous group is always easiest to design for. For example an aboriginal nursing home in Kalgoorlie, Western Australia can provide a log fire in the middle of the day room, and that makes sense for all the residents. A single aboriginal man in a nursing home in Northam may have to orientate himself to an environment designed for the wheat belt farmers.

Many units are intimidatingly posh for some residents. It must help to furnish single rooms with familiar items, ideally the resident's own furniture. Yet many rooms are kitted out with fitted furniture or there is no storage to allow the room to be emptied for the resident's own furniture.

Ethnic background is rarely taken seriously in design terms. In Australia many migrants will have spent their early lives in countries such as Greece and Scotland, yet the design of units tends to reflect early twentieth-century "Federation" Australian design. In the UK the same applies. Rarely are there design concessions to an Asian or Italian background, for example.

A home for life?

Whether or not a person with dementia is to remain in one unit until they die is a key issue in determining the design of units. We would all like to think that this is possible since it is certainly, at first glance, desirable. It is rarely

good for any of us to move, and moving someone with impaired reasoning can be very stressful. Having said that, many people with dementia thrive in a new environment if it better suits their needs. Sadly, the general rule of thumb seems to be that the more mentally disabled you are, the more disabling the environment provided.

Coon (1991) is not the only expert to stress that homogeneity of need is a determinant of good quality care for people with dementia. As we have said before, people with dementia are far from a homogenous group. At the most basic level people with dementia will vary in terms of their physical disabilities and will make very different demands on the environment in this respect, for example in terms of incontinence or mobility, or need for terminal care.

They will also have very different behaviours. Some people with dementia cope by walking great distances. Others can be extremely anxious and agitated and require to see staff at all times. Dependency scales, such as the Revised Elderly Persons Disability Scale (REPDS)**, provide a more rounded picture of the kind of dependencies which need to be considered.

The design implications of homogeneity or lack of it are many. A unit where people are physically very disabled may require space for hoists, drips, oxygen, etc. Space for sluices and for the storage of wheelchairs may need to be provided. On the other hand a home for people who have retained many skills and physical abilities, but have severe memory problems, may be more like an ordinary house. (Indeed, it may be an ordinary house. It is likely that over the next five years or so we will see a rapid increase in expertise in adapting or designing ordinary houses so people can remain in their own homes.)

People with high levels of agitation and challenging behaviours may need units where there are very high levels of visual access so they can see the staff at all times and the staff can see them. The issue of whether or not high levels of visual access are desirable for all people is unresolved. Yet it would seem sensible to design for the highest levels of disability in this respect so that people with dementia can increase their chances of remaining in the same place until the end of their life.

*Design for Dementia (ISBN 1 874790 35 3) is published by Hawker Publications.
**Fleming R, Bowles J (1994) How, when and why to use the Revised Elderly Persons Disability Scale. Macsearch, University of Western Sydney, Campbelltown, New South Wales.
• This chapter first appeared as an article in the Journal of Dementia Care 6(1) 15-17.

CHAPTER SIXTEEN
Just another disability 1: making design dementia-friendly

SALLY STEWART

Architect and tutor, Mackintosh School of Architecture, Glasgow

*T*hroughout 1999, as UK City of Architecture and Design, Glasgow became the focus for the European and international architecture and design community. As well as celebrating high profile projects, the year offered the opportunity to encourage links between architects, designers and the community at large. A number of significant projects were established to demonstrate the City's understanding of the importance of design and architecture in our lives.

One of the core projects set up to explore and celebrate the impact of good design focused on the disability of dementia under the banner *Just Another Disability: making design dementia friendly (JAD)*. The intention was that a series of connected projects and events would provide lasting benefit to the community by increasing understanding on how to design for dementia.

JAD was set up to bring together architects, designers, care professionals, people with dementia, their carers and families to create a comprehensive guide to making design dementia friendly. The project draws on good practice worldwide as well as the experience of realising three environments for people with dementia in the city.

People with dementia and those that care for them have been involved and consulted whenever possible to ensure that the hallmark of all the work is an understanding of the main users' needs and recognition of their wishes.

The project components

The project consists of a series of distinct elements. The elements are all quite diverse, each one chosen for the potential it has to highlight a particular series of issues designing for dementia brings with it, or to give examples of the difference good practice makes. The project elements include:

Development of a strategic brief

To provide an agenda for any architect or designer, or someone commissioning a project. At its heart is a series of methods of engaging with people with dementia as well as their carers and families, and assisting them to give their views and ideas to inform a design.

Development of an audit tool

To create a method to measure how well a home or centre fits the needs of a person with dementia. It can be used to examine existing and proposed buildings.

An advisory service

A telephone hotline offering design help to anyone who needs dementia friendly advice, and an information pack available from the project team.

A conference

An opportunity to discuss and share experience in dementia design prompted by the Glasgow experience, with published conference proceedings.

Customisation projects

Customising a house, a residential home and an acute admissions unit to deal with the problems of people with dementia.

Concept designs

Design models that anticipate the differing size and needs of homes for people with dementia in rural, urban and suburban locations.

Good design has a positive effect on everyone who encounters it. It helps the person with dementia to operate to their full potential and compensates for the disabilities dementia brings. Good design can establish a sense of individuality, promote dignity and well-being. Good design for dementia helps not only the person with dementia but their family and carers, and staff too. The vast majority of people with dementia live in their own homes, sometimes out of necessity where no alternative accommodation is available, but much more often out of personal choice.

Customisation projects

One of the live elements of the project was the customisation of three different living environments for people with dementia. The reasons for choosing a house, a residential home and an acute admissions unit were twofold: allowing the architects involved to examine the most common living situations of people with dementia, and recognising the extensive use of existing properties. The aim within each customisation was to produce a design template to be used by anyone in a similar situation to make their living environment dementia friendly.

A panel of architects was formed to work on the design of the customisations. While each customisation had a project architect, the panel worked together to develop and refine the solutions offered. As a method of working this is unusual, but led to a very positive dialogue between the architects involved, a collective sense of responsibility for the work produced and a much broader range of solutions considered. The progress and direction of the developing designs was discussed by the panel on a regular basis.

Crossmyloof Resource Centre

A large proportion of the accommodation available for elderly people with dementia is provided by residential and nursing homes. Crossmyloof Resource Centre is a typical example of a residential home built in the last 10 years

Crossmyloof is a two-storey, purpose-designed residential home for 48 residents, including respite accommodation, and a community day centre. The centre was opened as recently as 1994 and has a unit of 12 bedrooms on the upper floor of the west wing specifically designated for residents with diagnosed dementia. However, from the first survey and analysis, the design of the dementia unit does not differ in any respect from the other wings that are intended for physically frail elderly residents.

The project was designed to look at the current limitations of the design of the dementia unit and to suggest a range of alterations within a restricted budget. The aim was that the design should improve the quality of life for the residents and help the staff and carers to provide a better level of support and service.

Once the brief was refined over a series of meetings, preliminary proposals were drawn up and the group was extended to include a project manager, services and structural engineers.

From the original analysis of the building, several shortcomings in the design were identified that were contributing to a poorer quality of life for the residents and more difficult working conditions for the staff. The group identified the following significant problematic issues:
• insufficient space for lounge and dining functions at the same time
• no access to secure and purpose designed garden
• conflicts in use of kitchen by residents and staff
• inappropriate interior finishes and decoration
• bedrooms identical
• toilets not visible from bed positions
• dingy corridor and sitting area
• no quiet room
• no provision for dispensing of drugs.

Despite the building's limitations it is extremely popular with users and carers.

It was recognised that any extension to the first floor space would involve a commensurate increase in the ground floor non-designated accommodation. As a result of demand, the ground floor unit already has to accommodate residents with dementia but without the staffing benefits. The work to the first floor will therefore provide a future benefit in allowing an easy adaptation of the ground floor unit to bring it up to the same standard of dementia awareness.

Design solutions

At an early stage in the project two approaches to the customisation were identified. The first involved a radical remodelling of the layout to relocate the communal facilities close to the entrance to the unit. The bedrooms lost in this arrangement were shown added on to the far end of the wing. The second stayed with the present flawed layout and provided additional communal accommodation in a straightforward extension of the wing.

In terms of design for dementia, the former approach was felt to provide the better option but was not achievable in this exercise because of the strict budget limitations and the much greater disruption to residents' living conditions. The group had at an early stage in the proceedings decided that the option of total decanting could have a potentially serious impact on the more vulnerable residents and was therefore discounted. It was also recognised at this time that the construction work would have to be carried out in a way that would minimise the disorientating effect this could cause to the residents.

The remodelled unit deals with many of the limitations to people with dementia of the original design, within a limited budget and the restrictions of an existing occupied building. It should neither be seen as a stopgap solution nor a compromise, however. The design team was particularly aware that the unit was already the residents' home environment and that changes which would in the long term be therapeutic should not be disabling in the short term.

The remodelled unit offers the following measures:
• Existing bedroom doors are made more easily recognised, with communal areas redecorated in more appropriate colours and materials. Personal effects and memorabilia are used increasingly throughout the unit to stimulate memory and conversation.
• New skylights have allowed corridor spaces to be more pleasant, better lit places, without introducing disorientating shadows.
• Signage and handrails have been fitted where appropriate to help wayfinding, and encourage the use of all the facilities including a new multisensory room. Doors throughout the unit have been changed to provide an appearance appropriate to function.
• Within bedrooms toilet doors have been moved to allow the WC to be seen from the bed.
• More space within the living room allows all residents

to be seated, offering views to the street, to the garden, or the television or fireplace within the room. A permanent dining space provides a settled eating place and allows activities to focus on the kitchen.

• A new toilet directly off the dining/lounge area is easily accessible to residents and suitable for assisted use. Mechanical ventilation throughout has been enhanced to allow staff more control over air quality.

• Floor surfaces throughout the unit have been changed to allow non slip sections within wet areas, and plain carpet suited to shuffling.

• Improved access to and security in the new therapeutic garden to encourage its use.

This new garden has been created with access direct from both ground and first floors. This provides a safe, secure external space outside for the first time. Its design encourages walking and wandering, while plants have been chosen to stimulate the senses.

This redesign focuses on physical changes to a particular building to improve its dementia friendliness. Although staffing issues are not within the remit of this exercise, it was recognised that staffing costs in relation to the new layout would have a significant effect on the unit's sustainability

Construction work has now been completed, and residents and staff are growing accustomed to their altered surroundings. Initial feedback from carers and relatives has been very positive, and we are in the process of carrying out a formal audit to assess the impact the work carried out has had. We hope that these findings will inform any similar work carried out by the client in the future and form a model for designers working in this field.

• The work of the project can be visited at www.gsa.ac.uk/ architecture/JAD.

<table>
<tr><td>CHAPTER
SEVENTEEN</td><td># Just another disability 2: concept designs</td></tr>
</table>

SANDY PAGE & SALLY STEWART
Mackintosh School of Architecture, Glasgow

As a way of putting into practice some of the ideas generated and identified by the *Just Another Disability: making design dementia friendly (JAD)* project, an architects' panel was formed early in the project. Their main task was to produce designs that could be realised as live projects to demonstrate in a variety of settings and situations the potential for dementia-friendly design.

Although three case studies were identified in the public sector the panel was aware that it was going to be impossible to create customisations or new projects funded by the private sector within the limited time available. As private sector providers offer an increasingly large sector of the provision of care facilities for elderly people and for people with dementia, the group was keen to explore how the principles of good dementia design can be achieved within the framework of commercially viable schemes.

It was decide that a series of concept designs should be prepared based on current practices in the private sector tempered with speculative input from all those involved in the overall JAD project. Brian Gault of Young and Gault Architects was the panel member with extensive experience of this field, and he developed a series of solutions for this market.

Issues examined

The private sector is a major player in the provision of care facilities for elderly people and for people with dementia. We were keen to explore how the principles of good dementia design could be achieved with commercially viable schemes.

Private sector care homes built at present are very much constrained by costs, particularly costs of land, construction and staffing. Operators tend to have financial viability calculations down to a fine art and the present weekly allowance dictates that they can generally afford £4,000 per bed land value and £25,000 per bed build cost. For this nursing homes are very often built in 60-bed two-storey configurations and often in suburban locations where land is relatively inexpensive.

Although this model is the most commonly found in Britain, it sits rather uncomfortably in its surroundings, being neither truly suburban nor non-institutional in nature. Consideration of the particular needs of estab-

lished communities or their context is not normally the generator for providing such homes.

It was therefore felt that these issues should also form a major input into the way the concept designs were produced. This broader, contextual approach would hopefully provide more balanced models, which would allow discussion across the provider sector on a number of unusual yet important fronts. The creation of models firmly rooted in real contexts and using appropriate solutions for specific programmatic issues would also hopefully answer the need of addressing such provisions in a normal framework in a normal way. We were very conscious of trying to celebrate normality so the provision would take its place in the context as part of that context and not something imposed and outlandish.

Concept designs

Three different locations and circumstances were examined and solutions proposed for (a) a suburban site, (b) a rural site and (c) an urban site.

The suburban scheme

Many nursing homes are built in the suburbs because land is generally more readily available, and is generally less expensive than in the city. Many families live there themselves, and would prefer their parents/grandparents to be nearby. Staff availability and transport links are also generally good.

A typical suburban area would generally have a mixture of semi-detached or detached houses. A plot of land for a two-storey, 60-bed unit would need to be 1.2 acres minimum, or 2.5 acres for a single storey development. A fairly large footprint (building perimeter) is created with a single point of entrance and a large parking area to the front. Private gardens are to the rear, fenced in for security. With the best will in the world a building like this will always look institutional and instantly recognisable as such.

In order to integrate a care home into a suburban environment like this, we considered the principles of development in the suburbs. A private dwelling house in the suburbs with a front garden or semi-public space leading from the street was considered. The house is reached by a footpath, a driveway leads to the garage. Beyond the front door and beyond the fence to either side of the house is the private part of the dwelling. This arrangement is continued on either side of the road and a street is created.

The design of the suburban nursing home model uses the template of the suburban house to create a cluster of small, 10-bedded units or bungalows, independent but interrelated. Each has a front garden with a driveway and front door. A 10-person family lives here. The bungalow has an open plan kitchen, a utility room, bright and airy spaces that give access to safe and private gardens. Dementia-friendly features include a safe secure environment but with opportunity for personal space and quiet spaces. Orientation of the resident is assisted by the fact that there are no corridors and each space has interesting views or other features designed to make way finding easy without causing stress and confusion. There is ample space indoors and outdoors for safe wandering.

Key facilities are readily identifiable such as bathrooms, bedrooms and kitchen. Each single room has its own toilet clearly visible from the bed space. A homely environment is created by careful selection of furniture. The open plan kitchen, which has restricted access, is a focal point for most activities in this design as in a normal domestic environment. Where they are able, residents can perform daily tasks such as cooking, tea making, washing or drying etc. The building is dignified, non-institutional and domestic in style, and fits in with its neighbours.

Six similar units are linked together on a 2.5 acre site. Each unit has a separately accessed front door, its own address and each its own safe garden which can be laid out in different variations. Behind each of the private gardens there is a communal garden for safe wandering where considered appropriate. Differences in planting, gates and benches give cues for orientation and reference. The layout includes a central administration building or clubhouse, which could include community facilities such as day-rooms, meeting rooms etc. A private operator may decide to offer respite care or day care facilities.

The overall effect is significantly different from the normal 60-bed nursing home.

Could the private commercial operator afford to develop and run a facility like this? There are three key issues:
• **Land:** at 2.5 acres this is the same area required for a single-storey, 60-bed unit, therefore there is no cost impact. The more sympathetic appearance may be an advantage in certain neighbourhoods.
• **Build costs:** Build costs need not necessarily be any greater than a standard 60-bed unit, since the heating plant, kitchen facilities and laundry facilities are fairly domestic in scale, each bungalow being effectively one large family house.
• **Staffing:** If the GGHB Guidelines were applied then staffing costs would probably double, particularly due to night time care in six separate locations. With this in mind discussions were held with GGHB Nursing Registration Team and Social Services. Various options were explored including a 'spectrum of care' in which a mixture of trained and untrained staff could be used. A 'house mother' who would be responsible for both catering and laundry (presently unacceptable under guidelines) could be considered. There was a willingness to re-examine the rule book and on the basis that some compromises could be

made then it is possible that staffing costs could be kept within limits, which makes the whole proposal more commercially viable.

The impact of building regulations on the design of a development of this nature was considered. A meeting was held with Glasgow City Council Building Control focusing on issues such as travel distance, means of escape, areas of special risk etc. Due to the domestic nature of the building, it was generally agreed that there were no real difficulties in this particular layout. The fire officer was also consulted and a relaxation may be required on technical aspects of security and fire escape.

The rural scheme

We examined a live case on the Isle of Mull where the only privately operated nursing home had recently closed down. Elderly people requiring care now must leave the island for Oban or Fort William on the mainland. Due to the distance, families find it very difficult to visit and the elderly person's connections with the community are difficult to sustain. In isolation their deterioration becomes much more rapid.

On Mull there is a strong desire to create a development which keeps elderly people requiring care on the island and to provide a 'progressive care facility'. This is not a dementia unit as such, but begins to anticipate gradual changes in the needs of the resident, with dementia being one possible outcome.

The previous facility is adjacent to the cottage hospital and shares facilities and staff. This is an old prefabricated building and the elderly people live in fairly undignified surroundings. Before one site visit, a road traffic accident had occurred on the island. The accident victims were being sutured and awaiting transportation to the mainland while the elderly residents wandered in the same space.

A local association was formed to promote this project. It identified the need for 22 beds, mostly linked together. An easy solution would be a fairly large institutional building on the site. However, the success of this relies on its integration into the community and recognition of the local existing rural settlement pattern. The brief therefore for this development is for 12 very sheltered units and 10 nursing home beds of which two are for respite care.

Our response to this brief was to produce a development following a rural settlement pattern of small terraced bed-sit cottages along the B road that leads to Salen. Units with their own front doors and small gardens allow more able elderly people independent access. A further 'cottage' unit provides the nursing care beds and is linked to a community facility. This is rather like a village hall providing meals and a lounge for the residents but which can also cater for other functions. Other community uses could be attached to this such as a library (as in the Howard Doris Centre at Loch Carron), a hairdresser or visitors' centre. The cottage has all the same features as the bungalow illustrated in the suburban scheme providing a safe and secure environment but with links to the community unit to enable the residents to share in the activities and be totally integrated. As in the bungalow scheme they are easily supervised to provide a safe environment. There is a stimulating social environment. Anyone over 60 is encouraged to visit for meals.

The gardens are an important element here, since many of the residents probably have been crofters in the past. There is an opportunity to cultivate one of the gardens and to have free range chickens and other farm animals. Since the site is located on the gulf stream, a formal garden could contain palm trees and other exotic species common on the west coast of Scotland. This allows the opportunity for community involvement and integration into the community and the mainstream activity of the island.

The challenge is that circumstances here make any solution's commercial viability very difficult.

Land may be cheap but ground conditions are not ideal with a substantial amount of peat in the area. Build costs are expensive as all materials have to be imported by ferry. Staffing is also an issue, but if a similar spectrum of care is adopted as discussed earlier it may prove to be feasible. It is more likely to be viable however, as a joint venture between the Housing Association, Social Work and the Health Board.

We would argue, however, that even if the costs are significantly higher than the normal weekly rate it is a price worth paying to have elderly people kept in the locality close to family and community.

Urban model
There have been very few nursing homes built in the inner city areas, generally because land is more expensive. There are, however, many residential communities in the city such as the West End of Glasgow and the Merchant City and these are increasingly popular. Many people wish to be able to spend their later years in the same community in which they have spent their adult lives.

For the urban model, a high density site in the Woodlands area of the city was chosen. This is a tenemental area and an ethnically diverse community. The predominant building type is the four-storey tenement. Here the main issue was how to integrate a care facility for dementia sufferers into this environment both architecturally and socially.

As a key we considered how the Glasgow tenement operates. The buildings are accessed directly from the street via a close or shared entrance, with a stair well offering access to each flat. To the rear of the development is a back court area with communal facilities such as drying areas, bin stores etc. On the ground floor there may be shop units or commercial premises. We used this building type as a model for the dementia unit so it would fit into its surroundings.

With high land values, development on a site of this nature has to be either multi storied or include uses which generate high income. This was achieved by creating a lay-

out which included some commercial use such as shops or offices, a community facility, parking for rent and mainstream flats for sale or rent.

In the basement, parking (55 spaces) is provided for staff and visitors to the nursing home. The balance of spaces would be available for rental to local residents or for the adjacent business district.

On the ground floor, there are two independent 10-bedroom units containing the same facilities as those in the suburban scheme. As in the tenement these are accessed by a close and are effectively 10-bedroom flats, with a front door like any other. Once inside, the unit is designed to create a safe stimulating environment. A variety of day spaces give views over the street or views into and access to the garden. The garden layout in this particular scheme has been designed to provide a reminder of backcourts of tenement developments. The same stair gives access to the flats above. The building is set back from the street providing privacy, and daylight and ventilation to the car park below. A community facility provides meeting rooms and community rooms for functions. This could be utilised by the nursing home operator if required.

At first-floor level there are four separate semi-independent 10 bedroom flats each accessed from the close. The day spaces here also either provide views to the street or into the gardens and each flat or unit has access to the roof garden.

On the upper floors there are mainstream flats which are available for sale or for rent. Restricting the height of the east and west to two storeys allows daylight into the garden court.

This scheme allows people to remain in their community. The small units allow for an ethnic focus with distinctive interiors. The scheme doesn't look like a nursing home, it looks like an inner city residential/commercial development. It is an urban solution for an urban site.

In terms of affordability, a realistic land value should be achieved because of added value from the other commercial activities. The built cost will be slightly higher with the integration of stairs and lifts but this should be recoverable through the selling prices or rental values of the commercial and residential properties. If use is made of the same care principles with a house mother and a variety of levels of staff from care assistants to nursing staff, for each unit, as previously discussed, it may will be possible to make the whole scheme commercially viable.

Conclusions
As the private sector plays an increasing role in the care of our elderly population we hope that the opportunity will arise to translate these concept models into reality as permanent legacy of the *Just Another Disability* project.

Acknowledgements
Brian Gault, Young & Gault, Architects; Tim Sharpe, Joann Tang, Mackintosh School of Architecture; David Allison of Clyde Care; Ben Brodie of Carrick Care.

CHAPTER EIGHTEEN | Assistive technology in action

STEVE BONNER
Development co-ordinator, Edinvar Housing, Edinburgh

Almost without exception, the technology currently used in care homes is found in devices which monitor residents' activity. This is often technology of the most basic form – but there are many new devices and systems being developed.

The simplest technology found in care homes generally consists of nothing more than a pressure pad under a bedside mat, a weight sensing device under the leg of the bed or the mattress, a magnetic contact on a door, or a wire that is clipped to the resident's clothing and activates an alarm when pulled.

There is no doubt that these devices are effective, but they are of low intelligence, and some can and will be prone to false alarms. As an example, pressure pads on the floor can be set off by a book falling from a bed as easily as by someone getting out of that bed. By the same token, because the pressure pad is floor mounted, and because it simply consists of two pieces of foil with a piece of foam sandwiched in between, it can very easily be damaged by a heel, furniture leg or even a vacuum cleaner or floor polisher.

It is also important to consider the ethical implications of using devices such as clip-on alarms or bed/chair monitors. These effectively limit the movement of a person to the confines of their bed or their chair as surely as if they were strapped into it. Although these devices are used for the good of the patient, to prevent injury from falls, it could also be said that the equipment is used to reduce the need for care or nursing staff.

It should also be noted that such alarms are 'passive' – in many instances residents are incapable (either physically or cognitively) of operating 'active' alarms. Active alarms require the direct intervention of those who rely on them. Pull-cord or pendant alarm buttons linked to some form of 'care-call' facility (usually located in a nurses' station) are examples.

The problem with an active alarm system is that it requires a number of things of the user:

• **They are physically able to operate the pull-cord or pendant.** (They may be severely disabled, their injury or illness may have debilitated them sufficiently to prevent their use, or the person may have fallen out of reach of an alarm.)

• **They are mentally able to comprehend what the**
alarm does. (A cognitive impairment may prevent them from making the mental link between the alarm being activated and help being summoned.)

• **They have the cognitive ability to remember that an alarm is fitted.** (A cognitive impairment that includes short-term memory loss may prevent them from even remembering that an alarm is fitted, and indeed what it is for; also, the resident may be so distressed by their circumstances that they temporarily forget that the alarm is there.)

This isn't to say that active devices won't be used in a care setting, but in many cases they are likely to prove to be less effective from the point of view of monitoring safety and well-being, especially in the care of those with dementia.

Types of active technology

There is always a difficulty with the integration of technology into any building, especially existing buildings. This is even greater when considering a care home: incorporating technology while the care home is inhabited can lead to major upheaval and disturbance for the occupants. So it is generally better for this to be achieved while the building is being built – although there are schemes under development which would enable technology to be 'plumbed in' with less disturbance.

If the building is already in use, sometimes the existing technology infrastructure in the care home can be used (see below). The most obvious way is by using an existing care-call system.

Care call alarms
Manufacturers of care-call systems are recognising the need to expand the capabilities of their equipment beyond simple pendant and pressure pad alarms. Systems are now incorporating additional features such as movement detection (using a 'passive' infra-red sensor), fire detection (using heat and smoke alarms), door entry security, and even wandering and fall detection.

The benefits of using a system in this fashion is that it can be made flexible enough to suit the needs of a wide range of users. In effect, someone who is at risk from falls can have a fall detection monitor or a movement detector fitted, while if the next resident who occupies the room does not need these devices, they can be removed or deactivated.

Not all care-call alarms need to be 'hard wired' (ie connected by cables). It is also possible to use radio (RF) transmitters and receivers, infra-red controls and even 'mains-borne' signals to operate equipment. Mains-borne signalling is where the wiring infrastructure already in a building (usually appliance power outlets and walls sockets) can be used to carry signals to control equipment or transmit alarms. A common example of this in the domestic environment is the use of a baby monitors, simply plugged into a power outlet in the child's bedroom and the amplifier unit plugged into an appropriate power outlet where the parent is.

Door and door-lock controls

There is a range of devices which people with physical disabilities can use to unlock and open doors to permit entry/exit. On the whole these are too complicated for people with dementia to use themselves. They include double handles which are considered too difficult for most residents and, more commonly, devices which require a set of numbers to be punched in. Most people with dementia are unable to learn the numbers. Wrist watches and pendants which alert staff when certain residents go through external doors are increasingly common and can sometimes be programmed to allow residents access to their own rooms but not those of other residents.

Window and curtain controls

As with door controls, these devices are of particular benefit to those with physical disabilities. They are unlikely to be usable by people with dementia unless they have been using them for a long time – unlikely to be the case in care homes. It is possible that automatically operated curtains might help someone with dementia with time orientation problems. Curtains could open when it is time to get up and close when it is time to go to bed, which could help someone differentiate between day and night. For some people, however, there will be a danger that the sudden activation of curtains will be disturbing. This underlines the key principle that the use of technology should always be part of an individual care plan.

Environmental controls which keep the temperature or lighting levels constant have considerable potential if too much or too little heat or light is known to exacerbate a person with dementia's restlessness or agitation. An individual room can provide the optimal heat and light for a particular person.

Intercom systems

As well as door and lock systems, there is often a need to monitor who is coming and going at self-contained or multiple occupancy accommodation. This would require the use of some form of an intercom system.

There are two options, these being audio only or audio plus video. The benefits of video over audio are manifold, the main features being the ability to record on videotape who is calling, and enabling a person with poor hearing to see who is visiting.

For a person with dementia, again the difficulty is with control and comprehension. What happens if the image that appears on the video intercom or the television set is seen as other than what it is? A daughter appearing on the person's favourite television soap, for example?

Audio intercoms can be just as problematic, as a person might find disembodied voices very disturbing.

Fire alarms

A suitable fire alarm is a fundamental requirement for a care facility, and vital for any dwelling where a person with dementia lives. It will need to perform a number of functions:
• It must alert care staff when an alarm (smoke, heat, gas) is activated
• In the event of care staff not being on site, an alarm is communicated to a remote facility (care staff centre or even a relative's home)
• It must ensure that in the event of an alarm being activated, the supply to the cooking/appliances (electricity or gas) is switched off.

The one major drawback of a fire alarm being raised when there are people with dementia resident is that of the ensuing noise. An alarm that is audible to the residents/service users is not necessarily always the best option.

Toileting

There is a wide range of products available to assist in toileting and bathing, ranging from hoists through to 'sit-up' baths. An elderly, infirm or disabled person may be able to cope emotionally with needing assistance with their bathing, but in many if not all cases, the need to seek assistance with toileting is seen as a major loss of dignity and privacy. To that end, there are a number of products on the market to help retain that dignity and privacy; one product, the bidet toilet, is particularly well received.

The bidet toilet is a device that not only allows the user to perform their normal toileting functions, but will also hygienically wash and dry them afterwards. The only assistance they may require is with getting on or off. Another important feature is the fact that many models do look like 'normal' toilets, reducing the institutional feel.

Audible reminders/prompts

Buzzers, bells and alarms to remind people to perform certain tasks have been used for some time. The most recent advance in this area has been the used of recorded speech or computer-synthesised speech as the reminder. These devices can be used to remind a person to take medication, of an appointment, or even in extreme cases to urge them not to do something they are about to (eg leave the house, switch on an appliance).

The benefit of some of the audible reminders is that they can be recorded using real and if necessary, familiar voices. The disadvantage is that they are not suitable for someone who may be delusional, or who may become distressed by the sound of a disembodied voice.

Environmental controllers

These devices are used by any disabled person who is physically unable to operate any of the "active" technology devices already listed, plus a great deal of other domestic equipment (eg lights, televisions, computers).

These devices can be used in many settings, and a care home is no exception. Not only can they be used to operate equipment such as door openers and other 'assistive' technologies, but could also be linked to a care-call system to summon help in an emergency.

Relaxation and enjoyment

Technology can be life enhancing. One of its main functions can be stress reduction. Many care homes these days will have a multi-sensory room or multi-sensory equipment. These usually combine visual stimulation through attractive light and pictures, pleasant tactile stimulation, relaxing sound and sometimes even smells. The combination is provided to suit the individual as is the frequency and length of use. Less frequently used are tailor-made videos. They can combine material about the favourite places for that person with material about their workplace or hobbies. A lot of general television is meaningless to people with dementia. Local cable television may have more potential as it often shows local places and celebrations.

Touch screens may have potential for residents with dementia although their use is rare at present. They can allow people with dementia to make choices: for example, by touching the picture of their favourite singer, the person can hear the music they enjoy. Touch screens can also be used to provide simple memory games.

Conclusion

Without doubt, there is great potential for the use of technology both in formal care settings and the domestic environment.

The major drawbacks of the use of technology are that costs for some equipment are still high, it cannot always be easily integrated to provide a fully 'interactive' system, and the skills still do not exist to give care providers access to a 'system integrator' who can make the more complex items of technology work for them (and be readily altered to suit differing needs).

In a few short years we will start to see equipment that is fully interconnectable, is affordable, and will not be beyond the skills of a competent DIY-er or someone who is IT-literate.

No matter how the future shapes the advance of technology, we must not lose sight of the people it is there to benefit. The use of technology as part of a care package should be there to enhance the quality of life and ensure the safety of the service user. It should not be provided to replace the human face of care, nor to reduce existing care. Rather, it should be put in place to provide a better-focused, more appropriate form of care.

Further reading
Marshall M (2000) ASTRID: A guide to using technology in dementia care. Hawker Publications, London.
Website: www.astridguide.org